"*Yoga Therapy for Fear* deals with many of what I consider the most fascinating and important common-sense aspects of healing: breath, movement, trauma, fear, and how to assist others (and self!) in the unwinding of those internal 'not good enough' knots we all nurture and protect. A veritable cookbook of good ideas, thoughts and techniques."

—Noah Karrasch, Developer, Practitioner and Instructor of CORE Bodywork

"Reading about anger, fear, and all the emotions that are present in all of our lives, and seeing yoga therapy techniques that can truly make a difference has been splendid. I have gained so much, and know that this book can make a huge difference to so many."

—Sara Spoerri, Registered Nurse (RN)

YOGA THERAPY *for* FEAR

of related interest

Trauma-Sensitive Yoga
Dagmar Härle
Foreword by David Emerson
ISBN 978 1 84819 346 8
eISBN 978 0 85701 301 9

BodyMindCORE Work for the Movement Therapist
Leading Clients to CORE Breath and Awareness
Noah Karrasch with Robert White and Elizabeth Buri
ISBN 978 1 84819 338 3
eISBN 978 0 85701 295 1

Principles and Themes in Yoga Therapy
An Introduction to Integrative Mind/Body Yoga Therapeutics
James Foulkes
Foreword by Mikhail Kogan, MD
Illustrated by Simon Barkworth
ISBN 978 1 84819 248 5
eISBN 978 0 85701 194 7

YOGA THERAPY *for* FEAR

Treating Anxiety, Depression *and* Rage *with the* Vagus Nerve *and* Other Techniques

BETH SPINDLER

with Kat Heagberg *and* Kevin Richardson

SINGING DRAGON

LONDON AND PHILADELPHIA

Please see the copyright acknowledgements on page 12
for a full list of permissions granted.

First published in 2018
by Singing Dragon
an imprint of Jessica Kingsley Publishers
73 Collier Street
London N1 9BE, UK
and
400 Market Street, Suite 400
Philadelphia, PA 19106, USA

www.singingdragon.com

Library of Congress Cataloging in Publication Data
A CIP catalog record for this book is available from the Library of Congress

British Library Cataloguing in Publication Data
A CIP catalogue record for this book is available from the British Library

ISBN 978 1 84819 374 1
eISBN 978 0 85701 331 6

Printed and bound in Great Britain

FSC www.fsc.org MIX Paper from responsible sources FSC® C013604

My beloved teacher Eknath Easwaran set me on the course of realizing the depth of yoga, and understanding yoga and especially meditation as a healing modality. I wish to honor his memory always and encourage others to go to the source and read his wonderful words, through which he lives on.

Contents

Acknowledgments

I sensibly contacted the brilliant Kat Heagberg, Editor in Chief, yogini, and writer for *Yoga International* to spot me while I kicked up into the world of books. Her contributions are greatly appreciated, her work and suggestions impeccable. Much gratitude to *Yoga International*, from which I borrowed liberally as well.

And deep gratitude to my ever kind and patient husband, Kevin, who to my good fortune has lived his life as an artist/designer and agreed to work on the cover, photos, and illustrations. He assisted with all of my technical ineptitude and kept me fed and cared for when I was a bit too busy. Even my daughters, Emily, Paige, and Blythe, my husband and dear friends Sara Spoerri and Aurora Maxey consented to model for the many practices in this volume.

I am blessed to be part of a fantastic team who helped to create this book and to have access to some of the finest teachers in the fields of therapeutic yoga and psychology at my disposal.

The book is full of accessible practices that have helped so many of my clients, and I feel an urgency to share the work with others in the field of Yoga Therapy and related therapeutics to help us move beyond the world of "performing yoga poses" and instead open new doors for working in both a science-based manner and on a more subtle level as we practice ancient wisdom supported by modern research.

I hope yoga teachers and therapists will feel free to use the work presented here and to approach me with any questions.

Copyright Acknowledgments

Quotes on pages 39–40 from "Invocations to the Upanishads" and "The Rig Veda," as quoted in *God Makes The Rivers to Flow, Sacred Literature of the World,* selected by Eknath Easwaran, founder of the Blue Mountain Center of Meditation, copyright 2008, are reprinted by permission of Nilgiri Press, P. O. Box 256, Tomales, Ca 94971, www.bmcm.org.

Quote on page 80 is reprinted from Easwaran 2014 by kind permission of *Yoga International.*

Quote on page 82 from "Dialogue with Death," as quoted in *Essence of the Upanishads: A Key to Indian Spirituality,* by Eknath Easwaran, founder of the Blue Mountain Center of Meditation, copyright 1992 is reprinted by permission of Nilgiri Press, P. O. Box 256, Tomales, Ca 94971, www.bmcm.org.

Quotes on pages 197, 201 and 202 from *The End of Sorrow: The Bhagavad Gita for Daily Living,* by Eknath Easwaran, founder of the Blue Mountain Center of Meditation, copyright 1975, is reprinted by permission of Nilgiri Press, P. O. Box 256, Tomales, Ca 94971, www.bmcm.org.

All excerpts that have previously appeared in *Yoga International* articles are reproduced by kind permission of *Yoga International.*

Disclaimer

A reminder: The recommendations are intended to be general recommendations for yoga practitioners, Yoga Therapists, and teachers. They are not a replacement for the personal advice of a health professional.

Individuals at risk of stroke should exercise caution when adopting any inverted pose. For everyone, it is important to move out of an inversion slowly.

Preface

This book began when I was asked to review my friend's, body genius Noah Karrasch, excellent book *BodyMindCORE Work for the Movement Therapist*, published by Singing Dragon. I have written about yoga and Yoga Therapy for *Yoga International* for years and my fine editor at Jessica Kingsley Publishers, Sarah Hamlin, was kind enough to read my articles and approached me about writing a book on Yoga Therapy for Singing Dragon.

A glossary of Sanskrit terms is provided at the end of the book for those unfamiliar with them.

CHAPTER 1

Unearthing Fear

The Methodology

> **The enemy is fear. We think it is hate, but it is fear.**
>
> Mahatma Gandhi

The sniggering gargoyle perched on my computer. It hissed when I attempted to elaborate beyond a title. While I had published tons of articles about therapeutic yoga, yoga philosophy, biomechanics, debunking myths, and a little bit of everything to do with yoga, the beast jeered, "but a book?"

Even though I've practiced Yoga Therapy with countless people suffering from physical and emotional trauma and been a part of medical and psychotherapy teams that assist people in some of the darkest times, this fear demon insisted that a Yoga Therapist was not up to the task of writing a book addressing fear, deriding the fact that I do not have a PhD in neuropsychology and perhaps it would be best to keep the practices that I use, teach, and have found beneficial sequestered in the therapy room. But, because of the reaction I receive when I talk to students, groups, and clients about finding a path to courage and how it can affect their healing, I know that addressing this topic is needed by clinicians, therapists, and individuals wanting to delve deeper into helping clients and students recover from trauma and phobia, and that applications of yogic techniques can help us to live fearlessly.

How Fear Changes Us

Fear invokes wars, elects tyrants to government offices, sells cosmetics and medications, belittles the human spirit, and tells us we are not enough. Think about it. According to studies involving fear and loneliness by John Cacioppo, PhD,[1] we choose fear over trust nearly every time.[2] Keeping ourselves safe is a priority. We listen when someone warns us of the dangers of terrorists or impending disaster and tend to tune out compliments, kindnesses, and the brighter positive angle of a situation. We choose the candidate, the minister, the news that tells us how desperately at risk we are, rather than trusting in a system or process we truly believe to be good, life-affirming, or right. We tend to act from our own set of fears, defenses, conclusions, and desires to survive. Often, our reactions to circumstances are related to our past experiences, and in particular to the first few times that we experienced a similar situation to the one we are currently reacting to (usually something that happened when we were young).

Fear is addictive in that we seek out news and social media stories to reinforce our fears. Some households keep fear-based television news forefront from the time they wake up until they go to bed. We see clickbait images on our computers that upset or frighten us, but we can't resist the temptation to take a peek. We even enjoy (or think we enjoy) Halloween scares and gory movies as entertainment. It's that misguided survival drive that pushes us toward intentionally seeing if we are threatened. Margee Kerr, PhD, sociologist and author of *SCREAM: Chilling Adventures in the Science of Fear*,[3] states that "other 'feel good' chemicals can also come into play with fear, namely endorphins, dopamine, serotonin, and oxytocin: 'The neurotransmitters and hormones that are released are helping us prepare to fight or flee, at the same time our attention is shifting away from abstract thoughts and focusing on issues of survival.'"[4] It's as though realizing we aren't going to die produces a "natural high" and we become hooked on the scare. But we may wonder why we are tired. Feeling afraid exhausts the nervous system.

When we are frightened, the threat is perceived by the thalamus;* the stimulus is then relayed to the adrenal glands perched atop the kidneys, which go into overdrive, sending the adrenaline signal back up to the amygdala† at the top of the brainstem that we need to react (often in ways that would not seem rational to us in a more tranquil or resilient state). Our breathing and heart rate speed up, preparing the body to run away or fight. Blood flow is directed away from digestion and toward the big muscles of the extremities, enabling faster movement or the ability to hit or throw harder. The pupils dilate so that we can better see what is lurking in the dark. We may also freeze—the most primitive response of all—or hide from danger even, with the heart beating wildly. In fear states the hairs on the back of the neck bristle—for our ancestors this may have made them appear larger or more aggressive.

While a scary movie may trigger a jump or shaky reaction, we don't run away or strike out, because the rational mind can differentiate between real and fabricated danger; but the body is still cranking adrenaline and affecting every organ as though the murderous clown was waiting in the lobby.

But not all fear displays itself so blatantly as jumping, screaming, or bristling neck hairs. Our daily, more mundane fears underlie the three most daunting words in our language, "blame, shame, and should," and take their exhausting toll as well. These oppressive words can represent the fight, flight, or freeze response of the sympathetic nervous system and often on a less detectable, yet similarly exhausting and erosive way.

When we believe we are threatened, we blame others because we fear a differing opinion or can't bear to feel responsible for our own issues. If we can cast fault on another, there is some temporary relief from fear. Blaming is the "fight" response. We project the cause of our suffering and demonize "the other."

---

* A small structure within the brain located just above the brainstem between the cerebral cortex and the midbrain that has extensive nerve connections to both. The main function of the thalamus is to relay motor and sensory signals to the cerebral cortex.

† The tiny primitive amygdala is located in the temporal lobe of the brain and is the reason we are afraid of things outside our control.

Shaming ourselves and others is injurious to all involved and is a way of running away from our self-worth, fleeing from remembering who we are and honoring those in our lives. Shame keeps us small and binds us to repeating behaviors that seem safe but are actually harmful. Addiction is a prime shame response.

"Should" is the bondage we cast on ourselves or others to restrict and control. "Shoulding" is a freeze response: we hold our ground and disassociate from the present; we project an imaginary scenario on what has been done or what we believe must be done, from a place of inactivity. The "should" holds us hostage and in a place of judgment. In that land of "should," we see ourselves no longer in the place of fear, but somehow standing above or below it, stating how things might be done from a distance.

We avoid situations of uncertainty or present ourselves in costumes of habit to feel safe, but it's the experience of taking the job, risking the failure in a social situation, or standing our ground in the face of injustice that may be the greatest catalyst to our growth. What is it we are afraid of losing? The yogic sages had answers that ring true on a deep level. In Swami Madhavananda's translation of the *Vairagya Shataka* (*The Hundred Verses on the Renunciation*),[5] Bhartrihari describes how fear is associated with everything in the world:

> In enjoyment there is the fear of disease; in social position, the fear of falling off; in wealth, the fear of hostile kings; in honor, the fear of humiliation; in power, the fear of enemies; in beauty, the fear of old age; in scholarship, the fear of opponents; in virtue, the fear of calumny; and in the body, the fear of death. Everything in this world is fraught with fear. Renunciation alone stands for fearlessness. (Verse 31)

Author of "The 4-hour work week"[6] Tim Ferriss said, "What we fear most is usually what we most need to be doing." And unless that is standing in front of an oncoming train, it may be true.

Bhaya (fear) is considered by yogic sages to be a primary obstacle on the spiritual journey, though you will more often come across its more positive antonym in the ancient texts: *abhaya* (fearlessness).

Our path—physically, emotionally, mentally, spiritually, and in time—is ultimately determined by whether we continue in habit patterns of fear, or challenge those habits by forming new ones.

One might argue that normal instinctual fear is necessary to our very survival, as jumping from rooftops or eating poisonous plants is not a good idea for our species, and having rational fear is essential to achieve adulthood. But, some fears aren't supporting our survival. Phobias and aversions, such as fear of public speaking, feeling unattractive or an aversion to meeting new people, simply chain us to old *samskaras* (repetitive tendencies) and keep us wading through the same tired *karmas* again and again, and (according to the yoga tradition) likely lifetime after lifetime.

But if fear is the deepest of the deep in terms of being human, how does one root out such elemental stuff and maintain a strong survival instinct?

Yoga/anatomy teacher Leslie Kaminoff was asked in a classroom lecture, "How do you shift a *samskara* [deep habit pattern] that is generated from a bad childhood experience?"

Kaminoff replied:

> Make another *samskara*, a positive one that affirms your relationship to a universe that really wants to fill you with your next breath. *Abhyasa* and *vairagya* (consistent practice and non-attachment) is the advice in the [*Yoga*] *Sutras*. Connecting with the positive, disconnecting with the negative—they go hand in hand.[7]

But finding something that connects deeply enough to outweigh our negative tendencies may be a challenge since fear stems from something quite primal.

Neuroscientists have said for decades, "Neurons that fire together wire together." This means that while practice may not make perfect, regularly doing something helps strengthen the connections in the brain for that skill, and skills such as learning an instrument, speaking a new language, or establishing regular yoga and meditation practices are positive *samskaras*. Mindfulness, too, is a learned skill.

A very practical way to reinforce the brain's rewiring is by literally sleeping on it. If we are poking about on our cell phones (like we do) or watching irritating newscasts before sleep (yep, we do that, too), we reinforce the brain's connection to those activities. If, on the other hand, we listen to Brahms or read a book by Rumi or Eckhart Tolle, we enhance the importance of those activities. and memories in our thinking. The reason is something called glial cells[8] which garden and prune, especially during sleep, the least reinforced synaptic brain connections as though clearing shelf space for what we need. (This is also why that 10–20-minute power nap can make such a big difference in a muddy mind—we prune clutter during even short periods of sleep.)

This is a method of "making a new *samskara*," as Kaminoff recommends. Finding uplifting and positive input, such as reading, meditating, or using a *mantra* (a sacred phrase or syllable) before sleep. You can encourage your yoga students or clients to practice it, especially before they go to bed, and reinforce its importance during the day through words and actions, so these new skills don't get pruned. Taking breathing or *mantra* breaks or walks during the day, or picking up an inspirational read, can help with that behavior reinforcement and especially consciously reinforce what you want to retain before sleeping.

The process of changing old patterns of fear and addiction may take more than sleeping on it, though. It may take breathing through it.

To paraphrase a talk on fear and addiction by author/yoga teacher Rolf Gates, in an *asana*, or physical postures, class or Yoga Therapy session we can start addressing our fears as they come up via the breath, and rather than going back to old habit patterns, create new habits. He explains:

> Your first time in yoga class, when someone tells you to relax, you don't know what they're talking about, but you hear that 10 or 20 times and you finally take a breath and realize you can be in the same pose without holding the same tension… [You think]…I can start dealing with my fear as my fear and not your problem.[9]

But Gates says that dealing with fear is not an intellectual process. Our loops and patterns of fear are neurologically based. He affirms that they are most effectively dealt with via the breath and movement—our primary connections to the nervous system—and, according to author/researcher and psychiatrist Stephen Porges,[10] they are the main route to stimulating the vagus nerve, which we'll address later in more depth. When we take this route, over time, finally, the mind gets the memo.

It seems as though building these new patterns or positive *samskaras* should be straightforward: We see the good of it and getting better at life is the goal, right? Harvard psychiatrist Dr. Srini Pillay's study may indicate this to be a circuitous route. Pillay watched babies who were given a toy toss the object away time and again, only to cry at their loss until it was returned, then (you guessed it) throw it down once more. Researchers assessed this was a lifelong pattern. Humans are hardwired toward negative thinking and we notice the negative such a high percentage of the time, so we are more alert to danger. "We would rather master disappointment, than seek fulfillment," according to Pillay in a 2016 interview with Jon Assaraf.[11] This same rule applies to allowing fear to determine our choices and future.

Reprogramming the neural pathways of the mind toward fearless fulfillment, rather than seeking to master disappointment, is not something that happens to us or for us; it happens through us, and it requires a good deal of surrender—what the *Yoga Sutras* refer to as *Ishwara Pranidhana*. In that surrender comes the remembering of who we are: spiritual beings having a human journey (which we'll look at in Chapter 10).

Vedic scholars see the mother root of all fear as *abhinivesha* (fear of death). But why would standing before a podium, or requesting that a botched order in a restaurant be corrected, cause the gut clench of fear, as there is no risk to life there? What is threatened is the life of the ego. We fear humiliation because we identify more with the ego than our higher self, *Atman*.

The ego is perpetually afraid of its own extinction and will do most anything to stay untouched by change. It also has no room for love, because true selfless love overrides fear of death and has a drastic impact on ego. The parent or lover will not think twice about putting their own life in peril for the one they love. When I was sick as a child, I can remember my mother or father wishing aloud that they could take my illness and suffer themselves rather than see me with a high fever or a brutal cough. A comrade in battle will go back into the line of fire many times to rescue injured friends.

We may not even recognize fear in ourselves and others because it expresses itself so differently in individuals. The ancient science of *Ayurveda* has categories that help us make sense of why some might cower at a personal threat, while another despairs, and a third will resort to retaliation and violence. But they are all faces of fear, and whether life is threatened or our opinions are threatened, the brain reacts in the same way (more about that in a moment).

In an interesting study conducted by neuroscientists at the University of Southern California,[12] an MRI was used to see what area of the brain was affected by having one's political beliefs questioned. Researchers found that the affected areas were the insular cortex, which helps in decision-making and processing feelings, and the amygdala, largely considered "fear central" for the brain's activity. The study showed that when our beliefs and opinions are questioned, we feel threatened. Science has begun to investigate how meditation can positively affect these areas of the brain helping us find calm in the storm.[13]

Yoga asks us to let go of the idea that we are our physical bodies, our emotional states and, yes, even our tightly reinforced and guarded ideas about how the world works, as well as to let go of prickly notions about who we are based on a stance that may or may not be true; the reason being, it does not serve our path to become more self-absorbed, and we can be more effective as catalysts for good when we are practicing *vairagya* (non-attachment).

Now let us explore some therapeutic models for evaluating *dosha, kosha, vayu,* psychological condition, and stage in the healing process.

How Fear Exhibits in *Dosha* (*Ayurvedic* Constitution)

Vata (air/wind *dosha*)

We often associate anxiety with fear, and those of air/wind aggravation will most likely feel shaky, scattered panic when frightened. When one's small child is rushing toward busy traffic, the *vata* parent may alternately react with random striking at the endangered child or screaming hysterically and moving without thinking about the outcome.

Those who tend toward *vatic* provocation are also more likely to respond to a perceived threat with issues of loss of appetite, constipation, and shortness of breath. Remember, when endangered, digestion is less of a priority for the body, and breathing becomes rapid or retained while the brain chooses a course of action or escape. This is largely due to low gamma-aminobutyric acid (GABA), one of the main inhibitory neurotransmitters. When depleted, the brain gets stuck in hyperdrive and anxiety. And while all exercise helps GABA levels, one hour of yoga can increase GABA levels by 27 percent.[14]

Solid, grounding *asanas* with emphasis on connection to the earth and building strength help bring airy *vata* back to the earth (as opposed to dance-like *vinyasa* flow or rapid fiery breathing as in *Kundalini* Yoga, which may aggravate *vata* and cause problems with sleep).

Pitta (fire *dosha*)

Rage and anger are exhibited by those of a fire nature when in a state of fear. This pointed-blaming brand of fear is incited in times of war to invoke soldiers to fight and is also a primary tool used in elections. "Us versus them" is the basis of *pitta*-type fear. The fear reaction to a possible loss of a job might prompt cursing at one's supervisor or quitting before one has a chance to be fired. In an emergent context, the *pitta* versus *pitta* response often arises because no one is handling the situation correctly, and the outcome will be poor.

On a physical level, a *pitta* type will often experience elevated blood pressure, acid reflux, head pressure, skin inflammation, or fiery joint or muscular pain in response to fear. The *Indian Journal of Psychology and Pharmacology* posts that yoga practice is helpful for hypertension and elevated heart rates and that breathing-focused work may be of the most benefit for Type-A individuals with hypertension, as their breathing may be hot and rapid. Even extreme cases like choleric (*pittic* or "angry") schizophrenia have seen improvement with breath-centered yoga practice.[15]

Cooling breath practices such as *Sitali Pranayama* (slowly inhaling through a curled tongue and exhaling through the nose), or slow passive physical movement such as *Yin* or restorative yoga can help in the reduction of *pitta*-related symptoms and eventually lead to addressing underlying anger.

Kapha (earth and water *dosha*)

Imbalanced individuals in *kapha dosha* experience despair, depression, and hopelessness, or "*kaphic* fear." Tears and immobility, or heart-stopping frozen terror in the deepest crisis are also qualities of *kapha*. In an unhealthy or even abusive relationship, *kapha* will often stay and take it, and "numbing down" with drugs, food, or alcohol is not uncommon. The fear of change may even override the fear of physical harm.

Recent research at Boston University proved that GABA is a key player in lessening depression, and yoga was found to be superior to walking or strenuous exercise in helping with symptoms of both anxiety and depression as well as increasing GABA levels.[16]

Physically, a *kaphic* response to threat may involve overeating or oversleeping. Lethargy and lack of motivation to effect change may be present as well. In Yoga Therapy, empowerment breathing (expanding the chest like a superhero) and heated *kriyas* (outward actions to move energy) and *asanas* can be of benefit, as can breath work like *bhastrika* (bellows breath—forceful inhalation and exhalation) and *Kapalabhati* (Skull-Shining Breath—forceful exhalation and passive inhalation). (These are better defined in Chapter 11.)

Yoga can also reduce inflammation, which is a key factor in depression, rage, and anxiety.[17] A regular practice also increases levels of brain-derived neurotrophic factor (BDNF), a protein that acts like fertilizer for the brain, stimulating the formation of new brain cells; and new brain cells mean more likelihood of forming new habits and positive *samskaras*.

These summations are, of course, broad sweeps, and vary so differently between individuals, but are often good baseline indicators. We all have a mixture of responses to threat and they may change at different times of life or in stages of health.

A *Tridoshic* Manifestation of Fear

Recently, I was in rural Mexico, where I was hired to do yoga teacher training. After my arrival, I was informed that the training had been cancelled. I then had to find my way back to the USA around a holiday weekend, an impending earthquake, and a hurricane, and the person in charge demanded her deposit back.

I don't speak much Spanish, and figuring out how to get vegetarian, gluten-free food, safe water, and local currency was complicated. Getting home was much more complicated. To say that fear had not reared its head would be a lie. And in all its *doshic* manifestations!

I felt depressed (*kapha*) because I had been looking forward to this training and this trip, and was now alone (and unpaid as well). I felt anxious (*vata*) about my language barrier and lack of orientation; also, while walking through deserts and steep hillsides alongside rattlesnakes and scorpions in nothing but river sandals, I was less than protected. I generally have a good relationship with the natural world, but sometimes survival anxiety flares. And anger (*pitta*) was at a boiling point. I had been invited here and had taken over a month of time off (and lost a month of income) for a training that was now cancelled. This was definitely *tridoshic* fear, or a fear response pertaining to all three *doshas*.

So, what to do? For times like these, the common-sense therapeutic practice that my teacher Eknath Easwaran recommended was a *mantram* walk: taking a long walk while repeating a *mantra* in rhythm with your breath. If, like many people, you do not feel at home with a *mantra*, you can instead use a four-step breath focus (inhaling for four walking steps and exhaling for four). Some *pittic* types benefit from *sitali* (cooling) breathing—in through the tongue and out through the nose—especially in hot weather. *Sitali Pranayama* can be alternated with breathing through the nostrils in rounds as well.

This is one of the few yogic breath practices to use an inhalation through the mouth, which is specifically done to cool the soft palate and the area of the brain directly above it. *Sitali Pranayama* can be very calming and, as a prescriptive breath practice, is highly recommended in many traditional schools of yoga.

As a general rule, though, it's a good idea to breathe in and out through the nostrils. In fact, recent studies show that nostril breathing (just like the sense of smell) is connected to memory, and breathing through the nostrils can improve our recall.[18] When we are upset, our memory is affected, and a walk connected with a long inhalation and exhalation through the nostrils may help us remember more clearly, focus on the practical, and move away from rash, fearful thinking. Or, if we are prone to angry, resentful memories and that *pittic* manifestation of fear, the *sitali* breath may be especially helpful.

The walking helped me enormously, as did my daily practice. I also made new friends (*satsang*) and had the reassurance of not being alone. Never underestimate the company of like-minded people. A wonderful group of meditators and yogis took me in, even letting me teach a workshop to a delightful and eager group of people new to Yoga Therapy. Had I stayed in a brittle and bitter state of mind, I don't think I would have attracted comrades who helped me find my way across the border.

Coping with Fear via the *Panchamayakosha* Model

It's often easiest to see the physical effects of fear—dilation of pupils, loss of color or redness (depending on one's constitution), unsteadiness, or a furrowed brow—when worry or anxiety manifest in the *annamayakosha* (physical sheath, i.e., our body). Through the lens of the *pranamayakosha* (energy sheath), we observe changes in the breath as well as the startle reflex and in hypervigilance. The *manomayakosha* (mental/emotional sheath) spirals our thoughts and may lead us to believe everyone around us is aware of our inability to cope. Paranoid hiding actions and addictive behavior wedge themselves between the *manomayakosha* and our higher thinking at the level of the *vijnanamayakosha* (wisdom sheath). When addiction and paranoid behavior block our connectivity, we can't see the reasons behind life's circumstances or understand the passing nature of hardship or apparently frightening situations. We may attempt to reach higher states of bliss with addictive behaviors, but they only reinforce the spiral of fear and lack-based behaviors. *Anandamayakosha* is the layer of bliss that is revealed when the mind is calm.

An interesting facet of growth to a state of higher mind, which is at the heart of the *kosha* model, is that working through this process with layers of self is part of healing and ultimately evolution. Only very rare souls develop self-knowledge without the "dark night of the soul."

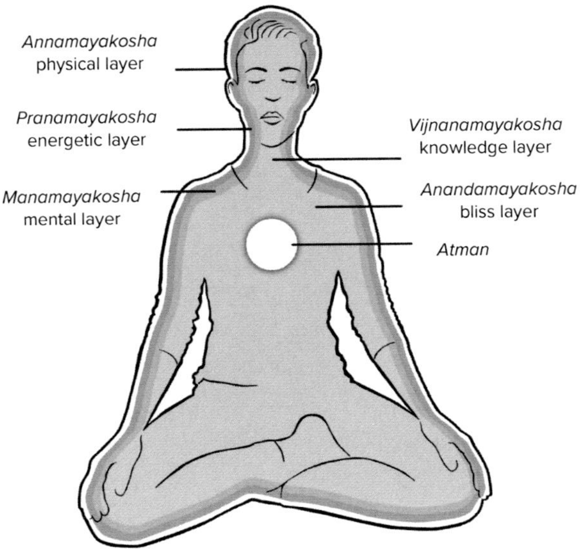

Figure 1.1 Panchamayakosha Model

The Role of the Yoga Therapist in Gaining Self-Awareness

The Yoga Therapist assists the client in working from outer to inner sheaths by starting with movement (no matter how subtle), which brings welcome ease and relief, I have never seen a person begin the process of *asana* and breath control without experiencing some level of positive change.

I realize I just used the word "process," and I have had to be careful with that and also with the word "processing," as in processing grief or trauma. After the sudden loss of her new husband, one of my clients told me, "I have no desire to 'process' my grief. Processing is what they do to food to take the life force out of it. I want my grief to be raw and real." I respect that viewpoint and see moving forward after tragedy more as a journey where we gain access to the recovery of our higher selves, with steps forward and backward and sideways. The journey is always organic.

Working with the *Pancha Vayus*

The *pancha* (five) *vayus*—also referred to as the *pranic* or *prana vayus*—are the dynamic winds in all of nature and in us, the energetic motions that are deeply affected by breath, movement, meditation and sound. When these *vayus* are in balance, health and well-being flourish; but when they are out of harmony, the use of yoga, proper food, and lifestyle changes can help re-establish equilibrium.

When a person has a tendency to take in fear via movies, news, or dangerous relationships, this is *prana vayu* feeding the fear cycle. *Prana vayu* doesn't make judgments or choose morally what a person "eats." They take in what is most readily available, be it bad food or good food, horrible ideas or beautiful ones, injurious sound or healing tones.

Developing a *mantra* or meditation practice to develop discernment (*viveka*) can be beneficial. Resensitizing the mind to turn away from damaging input is a major role of meditation. There are many types of meditation. Mindfulness or *vipassana* meditations cause the brain to rewire and become more sensitive to that which exists in the environment. In these more Buddhist styles, we become more aware of sensorial stimulation and thus we are helped to change our choices as to what we input and to be less judgmental about what life presents. On the other hand, inward-moving practices such as *mantra* meditation or contemplative prayer draw the mind inward and away from the senses, lessening the temptation to look for fulfillment in the outer world. While I have found both practices useful at different times in life, with clients I always start with simple breath focus and finding the sensation of stilling the mind. I let them choose what course they need—greater awareness of the world around them, or more interior time. Choice, for those struggling with fear or trauma, is one of the best tools a therapist has.

The inward spiraling digestive energy of *samana vayu,* which is not simply about intake of food, but of life itself, can be enhanced with *Brahmari* (Humming/Bumblebee) Breath and *Agni Sara* (Abdominal Lift) practices (see Chapter 10). Increasing power at the *manipura chakra* (navel center) can help a client build and create strength from deep stores. Gentle twisting and core-strengthening practices can also help heat the fire in the belly.

Apana vayu (downward-moving digestion energy) is often disrupted during times of anxiety (do you ever find yourself reaching for laxatives when you travel, or feel like you can't rest or sleep in new situations?). Digestion and elimination are aided by way of *asanas* such as strong standing postures, Child's Pose, *Apanasana* (Knees-to-Chest Pose), and grounding breath practices (balancing *apana vayu* is especially valuable for *vata* and *pitta* provocation). (See Chapter 10 for a whole practice to deal with bloating, gas and constipation.)

Vyana vayu (expansive energy) in excess can manifest as constantly changing jobs, moving unnecessarily, taking health risks, or frantically seeking help. *Vyana* deficiency, on the other hand, can cause a fearful person to isolate themselves. Breathing and meditation practices that assist circulation and cultivate a sense of radiance (see Chapter 12) with more rapid alternate nostril practice, such as *Surya Bhedi,* can help balance *vyana vayu* in both directions, both when it is in excess or in deficiency, as when a person is wound in on themselves. The deficiency can be observed physically, as in slumping and binding up arms and legs when seated, or in the emotional inability to see out of the depressed state.

Udana vayu (upward-moving energy), which often moves via the throat, can be obstructed in times of fear and the client may avoid talking. In such cases, vocalization such as humming or yelling, Hand-to-Heart *Kriya*, and chanting can be balancing. Interestingly, the same practices can help with the desire to over-talk or obsess on one subject. These practices help regulate the flow of upward-moving *prana* (life force or that which sustains life).

HAND-TO-HEART *KRIYA*

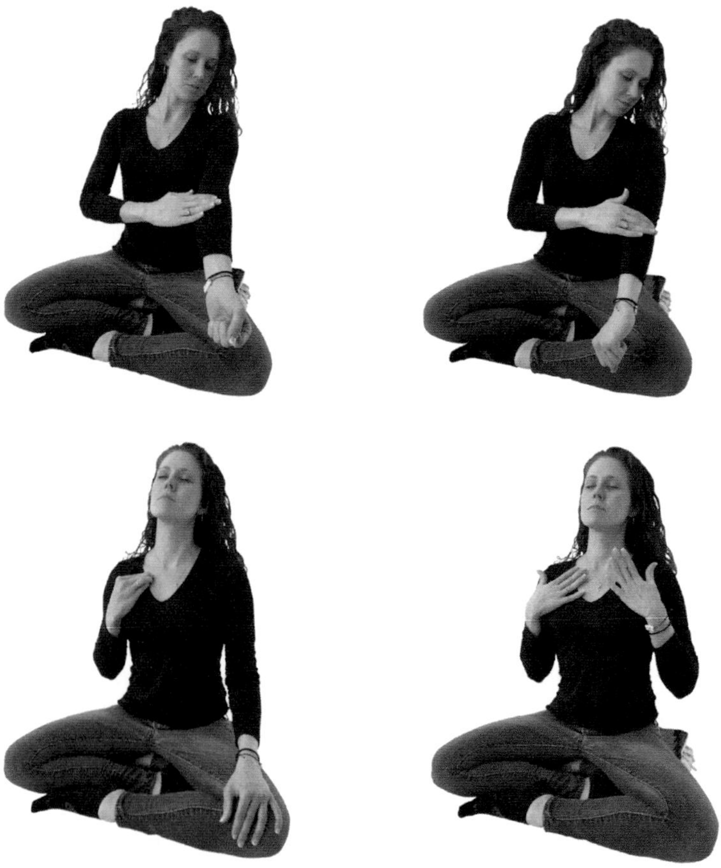

Sit upright, taking your right hand and tapping up the inside of your left arm from your hand, and down the outside all the way from your shoulder. Inhale as you tap up, and exhale as you tap down. Do 4 rounds up and down. Switch to right arm tapping and do the same action. Then make a small cluster with your fingers and tap just to the left side of your chest wall (look out for a light fluttery sensation in your chest). Now expand your hand and keep patting. Next, using both hands, pat your whole chest. Finally, let go of your voice with an "ahhh" sound (a little like Tarzan). Do that 3 times, then rest and notice how you feel.

Psychological Conditions

In my work with individuals in rehab and recovery, as well as those who are incarcerated, I come across many people who have experienced an overwhelming amount of abuse and trauma. Often, I've seen that yoga positions that one would normally do in a public class can be triggers for anxiety, and as a result, I've had to adapt my approach. A therapist must change their approach when they suspect trauma as a factor. But we must also keep in mind that we may not have any idea whether or not a student or client has experienced significant trauma, because many people are not able or willing to talk about their trauma at all. Therefore, I recommend assuming that everyone we work with may have been psychologically injured and be moving very gradually into what may be "trigger movements." I'll go into trauma-sensitive yoga in more detail in Chapter 6.

If we are endeavoring to look at our work from a holistic point of view, psychological factors cannot be separated from *doshic* issues, as *kapha* underlies depression, *vata* underlies anxiety, and *pitta* triggers anger. Helping to balance the mind with appropriate breath, movement, and lifestyle has an enormous impact on diagnosed conditions, and many psychologists and neurologists are exploring *Ayurveda* and yoga's impact on trauma and dysfunctional adaptation.

Stages of Healing and Individual Approach

No matter how injured or ill we are, there is always mending going on. It is the nature of being alive to heal. So, those of us working in the field can look at wellness as a spectrum, rather than a state.

At what point does Yoga Therapy enter the picture? This depends on the experience of the therapist/teacher. Many times, a referral to someone who knows more is in order. I call this the "Billy Goat Gruff method": "Don't use me! Use my teacher, who knows more about spondylosis or addiction." Scope of practice is an easy thing to overlook when we just want to help. We need to listen closely to those who come for help, and ask ourselves if someone else can better serve the person in front of us.

Does the client have a dianosis of early-stage Parkinson's and is not yet experiencing many symptoms, or are they dealing with serious mobility and stability problems and the concerns about moving about daily? Are they through with chemo and in remission from cancer, or are they trying to decide a course of treatment? Has it been 6 months or 20 years since the death of their sister? Yoga Therapy can enter at any point on the continuum as long as the therapist has training and experience in the issues of the client.

A therapist also needs to vary their approach, depending on a client's relationship to yoga itself. Someone with a history of being hurt in a yoga class is going to require a different quality of attention than someone who has taught yoga themselves or, conversely, someone who has never tried yoga at all. Emotional reactions, whether to yoga itself or to private therapy, may be rooted in past experience, and sensitivity to the client/student's resentments may determine whether the work in yoga continues or not.

The resentment/forgiveness factor, as well as the therapist's approach, can play a large role in a client's willingness to move toward healing. Many modern psychologists are warning against a therapeutic approach that is too compassionate or mothering as this may be a trigger for someone who has experienced betrayal at the hands of someone they trusted. So some personal distance and detachment may be in order for the Yoga Therapist as well.

Resentment can be the primary impediment to personal and spiritual growth, and it can undermine our courage. Resentment, while *pittic* in nature, is suffered by all of us at various times in life.

While we may have overcome addictions to alcohol, prescription drugs, food, sex, gambling, etc., there is often another shoe waiting to fall. The Big Shoe, Resentment! The big heavy snow boot at the base of all the addictions, and frequently a result of trauma and the resentment of what's happened to us. It's a source of recurring pain that can cause the desire for numbing, shutting down, or escape.

This process can actually be a gift, one we both give and receive: letting go of resentment. Truly letting go means no resentful words, no hard feelings, no jealousy, no self-righteousness, no coveting, no anger. Easwaran defined anger as "dwelling on negative thoughts, nothing more."[19] We may not be able to control the negative thoughts coming up, but by choosing not to dwell on them, we can take away their nourishment and the TLC that we have so lavishly bestowed to encourage their growth.

The greatest gift that we can give to both ourselves and others is one of omission, the omission of resentment. The absence of so large a *samskara* can create a home large enough in which to grow and thrive, and gratitude is a mighty ally against feelings of resentment.

Gratitude Practice as a New *Samskara* to Replace that Old Habit Pattern of Resentment

I was recently asked to present a weekend workshop on gratitude. I accepted the invitation—and then panicked. In my first wave of panic, I felt grateful that at least I hadn't been asked to do a weekend's presentation on geometry even though this invitation seemed nearly as far out of my wheelhouse.

Isn't thankfulness a sticky, smarmy, holiday kind of thing that cheerful, "everything is hunky-dory" folks do? Anyone who has sat in my teacher training classes knows of my penchant for satire and snark, and for debunking tightly held darling notions. But as is often the case, we end up teaching what we most need to learn—and it turns out that I'm more of a grateful-nik than I thought.

These are important things that I recalled and tried myself when preparing to teach the workshop on gratitude and transforming our thinking. I hope you find them useful for yourself and students.

Less is more: Minimalism isn't deprivation

Take a look at how our palate changes when we reduce sugar, spice, or salt for a time. When we reintroduce one of these to the diet, the flavor becomes intense—too sweet, too salty, too spicy. The same is also true in the reverse—for example, when we wear headphones to listen to music, we shout to compensate for being unable to hear over the excess sound in our ears. As another example, Leslie Kaminoff (the yoga teacher/anatomist I referred to earlier) likes to point out that when the feet can't feel the earth beneath them because of dense soles and structured shoes, our feet have to strike the earth harder to gain the same information. With excess, we need more input. Sometimes feeling afraid is something we add to our day, to feel more.

In terms of gratitude, this means that if we become accustomed to finding satisfaction from doing and owning more, it will likely take more and more stimulation to attain the same level of positive feelings. While no one would advocate for intense suffering and deprivation as a means of feeling grateful for any good that comes along, owning four pairs of boots may really not engender more positive feelings than one great pair.

The same could be said of having five yoga certifications or making dozens of pilgrimages. More is simply more. Caring more for what we have right now, and less about what we lack, is a key to happy living and encourages less fear of loss.

It is in giving that we receive

We know that generosity and service make us feel better. But according to Stephen G. Post, PhD, Professor of Bioethics at Case

Western Reserve University School of Medicine, altruism can also grant us a longer life.[20]

We all know the "feel-good" moment of sharing abundance with someone less fortunate. St. Francis may not have known about endorphins, but he knew much about the beneficial effects of gratitude. We receive from giving, and one of the things we receive is boldness. Knowing we have something to give helps us to feel worth, and shame and lack of worth underlie much of anxiety and depression.

Weed out complaints

We're often inclined to amuse ourselves with recounting our misfortunes rather than the smiles and sweetness in our day. Becoming aware of that tendency can help us focus more on the positive. My friend, author and minister Will Bowen, wrote the book *A Complaint Free World*, advising us to recondition ourselves to positive speech. Using a simple bracelet, we simply move it from one wrist to the other each time we hear ourselves complain—calling our attention to our *samskara*. The goal is 21 days of complaint-free living—which is tougher than you might think. But this intentional weeding works in us, as in all areas of nature. (Remember those glial cells that prune the lesser-used neurons?)

Little reminders

Giving the mind daily post-it notes is a way to encourage the brain to think fewer anxious thoughts, and less randomly, and to be more careful about what we choose. Remember that neurons that fire together, wire together, which means that repetition strengthens brain synapses. Daily practice, or *sadhana*, enhances our ability to stay positive and grateful throughout the day—particularly if done with affirmative and heartening focus. Repetitive gratitude practices, whether written or recounted mentally, are tools for becoming better at life.

One way to keep your focus on the positive is gratitude journaling. My husband and daughters produce gratitude journals in exquisite script, rendering frameable illustrations in the margins. I do not. My handwriting is more erratic than that of most fourth-graders, and I scratch out unwanted words vigorously—which does not make for a pleasing presentation. Sometimes I journal on my computer (with some entries becoming nice posts for social media—though that's not really the goal), or I just keep my scribbly words to myself in tea-stained, bathtub-wrinkled, spiral-bound notebooks. Making a habit of gratitude is what matters, whatever form your journal takes. Remembering the good in our lives helps us reprogram the fearful mind.

The company you keep

Another fine way to reinforce our brain's positive connections is through human connection. Spending time with people who help others and live lives of gratitude can help us see gratitude as a normal daily behavior. If instead we hear complaints all day, we become conditioned to see complaint as the norm. If friends who reinforce a norm of gratitude are rare in your life, look to the sages. Memorizing short passages from great teachers, and then recalling them throughout your day or in meditation, is a gratitude magnet. I offer the following passages as powerful reminders to be grateful:

> May I open my eyes in the morning with the Holy Name on my lips.
> May I see Divinity everywhere and in everyone.
> May I never hurt anyone and may I never be afraid of anyone.
> May I be inspired to choose persuasive words,
> loving language, creative and positive thoughts
> to bring peace and goodwill throughout the world.
> May my meditation deepen so I can draw upon the Source of all life for healing myself and the world.

> May I fall asleep at night with the Holy Name on my lips, healing my wounds and preparing me for another day of service.

From The Upanishads *(Translated by Eknath Easwaran)*[21]

> Breathing in, I calm body and mind. Breathing out, I smile. Dwelling in the present moment I know this is the only moment.

From Being Peace *by Thich Nhat Hanh*[22]

Every day, think as you wake up:

> Today I am fortunate to have woken up.
> I am alive, I have a precious human life.
> I am not going to waste it.
> I am going to use
> all my energies to develop myself,
> to expand my heart out to others,
> to achieve enlightenment for
> the benefit of all beings.
> I am going to have
> kind thoughts towards others.
> I am not going to get angry,
> or think badly about others.
> I am going to benefit others
> as much as I can.

Dalai Lama

> God makes the rivers to flow. They tire not, nor do they cease from flowing. May the river of my life flow into the sea of love that is the Lord. May I overcome all the impediments in my course.

> May the thread of my song be not cut before my life merges in the sea of life.

> Guard me against all danger, O Lord. Accept me graciously, O King of kings.

> Release me from my sorrows, which hold me as ropes hold a calf. I cannot even open my eyes without the power of your love.
> Guard us against the grief that haunts the life of the selfish. Lead us from darkness into Light.
> We shall sing of your love as it was sung of old. Your laws change not, but stand like the mountains.
> Forgive me all the mistakes I have committed. Many mornings will dawn upon us again. Guide us through them all, O Lord of Love.
>
> *Rig Veda*

A few years ago when making a move across the country around Thanksgiving, I wrote these words, which still hold true for me:

> Not preaching, just working on this myself;
> On Moving out of State.
> Gratitude is a state, so is peace of mind. Missouri is a state as well, Pennsylvania, California. We know they exist because we've been there.
> If I were planning to make a major move or even take a trip, the most essential thing I'd do would not be rent a truck or get gas. the most essential thing is to leave the place I am right now. Not with grudges or without understanding what I learned there, but with a willingness to put miles between myself and where I am now.
> So if I am going to a place of Peace of Mind I must leave the state of War of Mind. If I am going to live in gratitude I must completely leave the place of "Why me?"
> Blessings to you on this day of honoring a state of gratitude. May we pack lightly and move there with everything we need stored safely in our hearts.

It is simple in theory, isn't it? Reinforce your brain's "gratefulness receptor" with reminders in written and spoken word. Discourage your whining through self-observation. Seek the company of the grateful, learn to live minimally, and care about the little things.

Becoming a grateful-nik is not an overnight makeover. But you'll soon see that the flow of energy released by gratitude can both enrich our own lives and serve all those we meet.

Addressing Fear Following Betrayal

We may feel deceived by a betrayal of relationship, such as a marriage or friendship, a job loss, or a betrayal of our own bodies. For example, we try to do the right things to maintain good health and yet still experience health issues like a heart attack, a stroke, or osteoporosis. We have given our best and received what appears to be punishment.

Some of life's hardest blows are the end of a long-term relationship or career, or a negative diagnosis for ourselves or someone we love. When we feel deeply betrayed, it's okay to feel mad and even afraid about that. But the steps that we take after and during that initial angry, anxious, depressed time are important. Sometimes the feelings of betrayal last years, even lifetimes. The task is to find ways to dissipate the self-destructive element so that it isn't a fire that burns us physically and mentally. When we experience betrayal and feel panic or despair, it can be tempting to anesthetize the experience (which, generally speaking, is probably not the best long-term solution!), but I am NOT meaning to imply that prescription medications are never beneficial or appropriate or that someone should ignore the advice of their healthcare provider or feel ashamed about taking them.

The practices given in the *Spandana* section (see Chapter 6), while not a panacea, are great for working through emotional challenges or the daily chaos we often accept as the norm. It takes the deeper practices of meditation to truly work at the roots of feelings of being cheated by life.

Fear in the Bones

When it seems the body has betrayed us, it can shock us to the core. My first diagnosis of moderate osteoporosis occurred in my early 40s. This was after being besieged with tests, with monthly iron infusions for nearly 10 years, and treatment for B12 and folic acid deficiency. Finally, the osteoporosis and an intestinal biopsy pointed to severe celiac disease (extreme gluten sensitivity). After that diagnosis, I continued a very strong *asana* and walking practice and taught many teacher trainings. My diet changed drastically. Since then, I have led a gluten-free life, which requires me to practice diligence and extreme caution in order to avoid even minor dietary cross-contamination (like avoiding the gluten-free pizza in a restaurant where wheat dough is thrown in the air, forgoing a gluten-free cookie on a tray shared with other cookies, and finding a bit of humor when people suggest I "just pick the croutons out!"). It's a really strict thing, an autoimmune disease, not an allergy, and I had been doing everything "right," only to find out that in my late 50s, I have advanced osteoporosis with medical warnings that lifting a gallon of water could cause a fracture. Betrayed and afraid? Yes, I often feel that my strong body betrayed me, but I know the mechanics of the body and intend to keep my practice, though perhaps in a different way than my teachers originally taught. And for that matter, I will also lift gallon jugs and carry my laundry, just with more awareness to spinal care.

When clients come to me with bone or disc issues, I often sense a good deal of fear about movement, but they can benefit most from yoga's many boons as well as other physical activity. The fear stems from the idea that what they have is irreversible and will only get worse. It takes time and care as a therapist to build confidence that there are things they *can* do and that will help them in their strengthening process to help support their alignment and live with less pain and anxiety.

First off, the best ways to avoid fracture in *asana* if you have bone loss is to avoid jumping, pushing deeply into twists, rounding up or down into Forward Fold, "rock and rolls" (rolling back and forth on the spine), or rolling into Plow or Shoulder Stand, and bearing weight on the head in Headstand. Wow, that seems like a lot of "no" yoga, but there is plenty left for you or your client to practice!

A GENTLE, FEAR-FREE PRACTICE FOR OSTEOPOROSIS OR DISC ISSUES

Many of the options in this practice are excellent for those who have been diagnosed with a disc herniation as well. It's important to regain trust in our bodies. These movements feel good and strengthening, and help us feel more confident in daily movement. Your props will be a chair, a bolster, and a block, and maybe a blanket for cushioning your upper spine in the hip-supported inversion.

NECK AND UPPER BACK STRENGTHENER

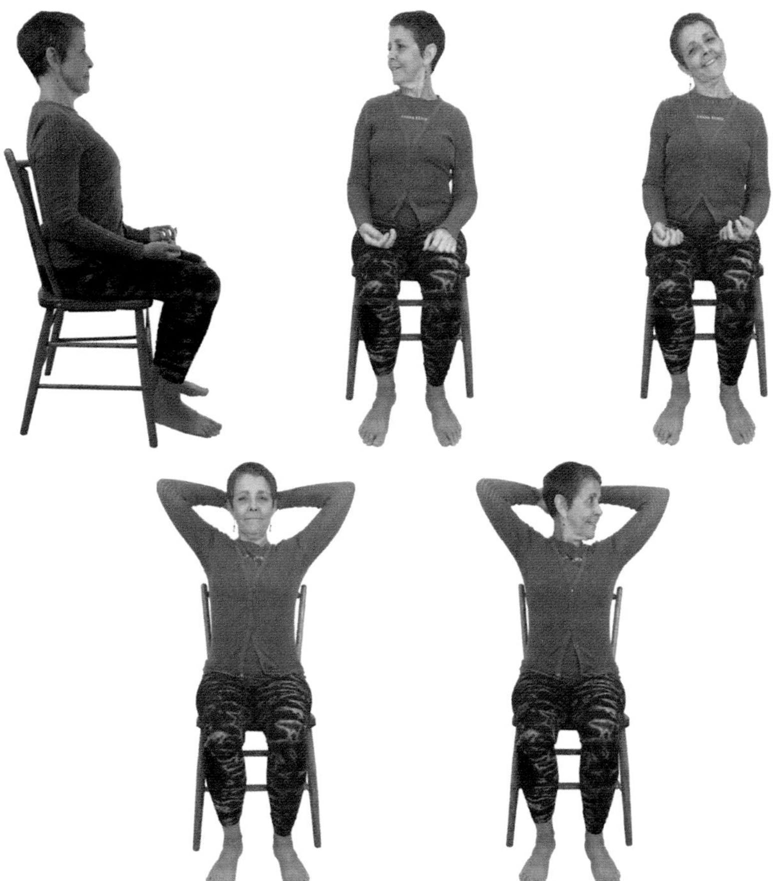

Begin seated in a chair with your spine tall. Envision drawing your head up and back and then extend your neck upward. From that centered position, turn your head to the right on the exhalation. Return to center on the inhalation, then exhale and turn your head to the left. Avoid pushing your face forward on the pivot. From center, with your chin slightly tucked, on an exhalation, move your right ear gently toward your right shoulder. Inhale, return to center, then move your left ear toward your left shoulder on the next exhalation. Inhale and return to center. Repeat.

Then, still seated, interlace your hands behind your head and press the back of your head into your interlaced hands and think of lengthening the back of your neck. Then turn your head to the right, press the side of your head into your interlaced hands on exhalations, and do the same on the left. Repeat 3 times.

SAFER TWISTING

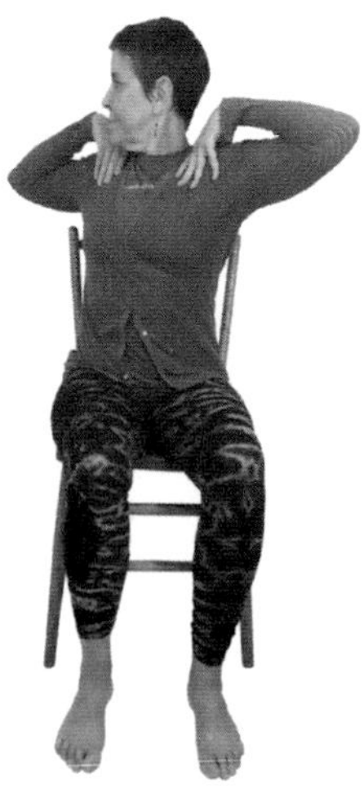

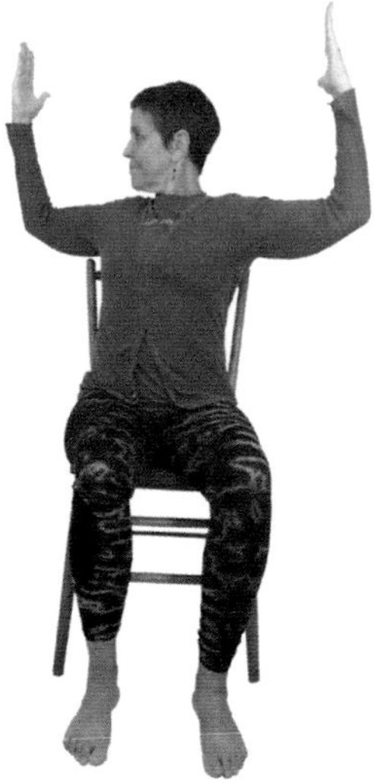

We are prone to overdo a twisting pose when we leverage into it by pressing with our arms and hands (often while keeping the core relatively passive). The secret is to engage the obliques to support the twist and to work at only 20–30 percent of our revolving capacity. In this way we are providing axial extension and helping to protect our bones and discs.

Still seated in a chair, place your hands on your shoulders and lengthen your spine. On an exhalation, turn your heart to the right, lightly contracting your abs as you pivot but still keeping your spine tall, making the twist a core-strengthening and shoulder movement rather than a lumbar spine torque and tug (the lumbar is where most spinal fractures occur with bone loss). For variation try taking the arms to "goalpost" or fully extend them out to a "T." Revolve on the exhalation for 3 rounds and hold on the last for 3 breaths.

CHAIR-SEATED FOOT STRETCHES FOR BETTER BALANCE

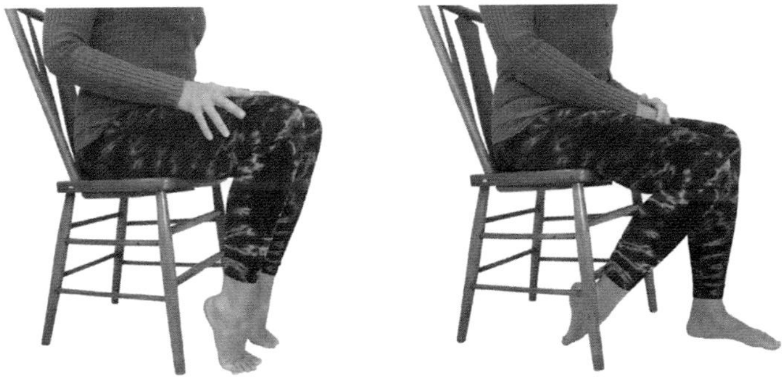

From seated, with your feet flat on the floor, lift your heels to come into a high tiptoe position, as though you were wearing Barbie's high heels. Hold for 2 breaths, lower your heels to the floor and then stretch the tops of your feet by placing the top of your right foot on the floor (toenail-side down). Stay for 2 breaths and then repeat on the left side. Follow this by tapping your heels rapidly into the floor then tapping your toes. The idea is to wake up the proprioceptors in the feet, which can be helpful for avoiding falls.

STANDING FOOT AND ARCH STRENGTHENERS

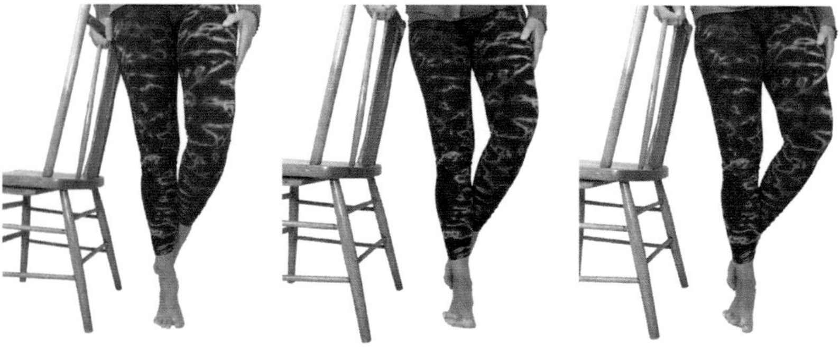

These are great for strengthening the arches of the feet and for developing ankle stability.

You'll do these standing on one foot. You can hold onto a chair for support. Come to stand on the inside foot. If you like, you could wrap the lifted foot behind your standing-leg calf. Inhale, rise up onto the ball of your standing foot and then exhale, and lower back down. Do 5–10 lifts. Use the whole ball of your foot for support. Then bring your whole foot solidly to the floor. Imagine your foot as a circle and swivel on it clockwise four or more times and then counterclockwise with your other foot still lifted. See how much more connected and strong that foot feels after you ground both feet. Now do the same on the other side.

SPARROW POSE

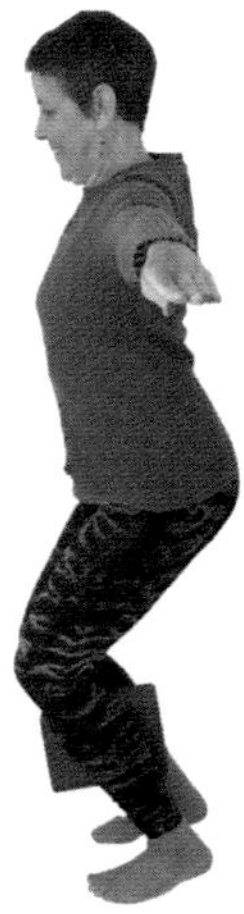

This pose engages your adductors, strengthens your feet, and strengthens the muscles supporting your lumbar spine. Place a block between your shins (narrow to mid-width) and bring your arms straight out to a T position. Keep your heels on the floor for the first couple of shallow squats, so you get the idea of maintaining a neutral spine, with the same natural curves you have in your back when you're standing upright. Then try to lift your heels as you squat down to a comfortable level (no deep squats, though, just Chair Pose level). Try working up to 5 squats and hold the last squat for 3 breaths.

LATERAL SPINE STRENGTHENER

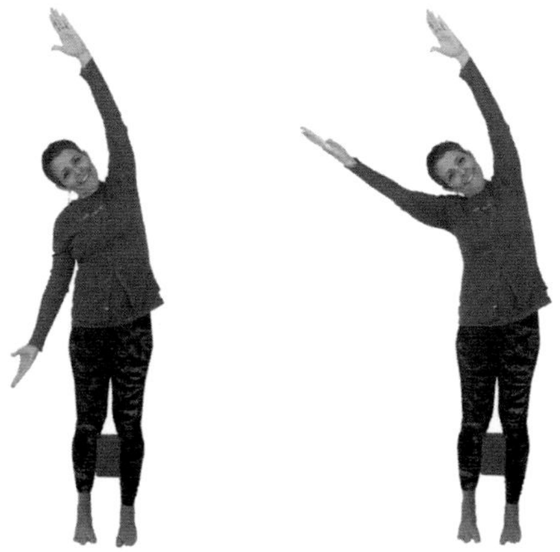

Keeping the block between your shins and both feet grounded, exhale as you slide your right hand down the side of your body, reach your left arm up on the inhalation, and gently arc to the right for 3 breaths. Inhale, lift your right hand up to join the left 3 times exhaling as you lower it down, and then hold at the top for 3 breaths. Inhale, return to center, lower your arms for a few breaths, then repeat on the other side.

CHAIR-SUPPORTED SUN SALUTE

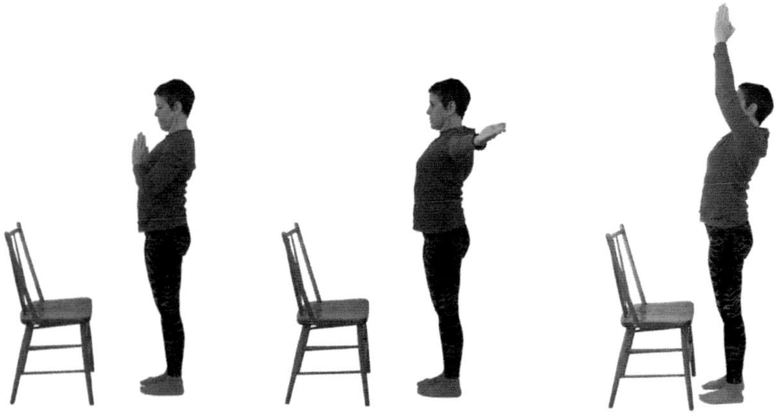

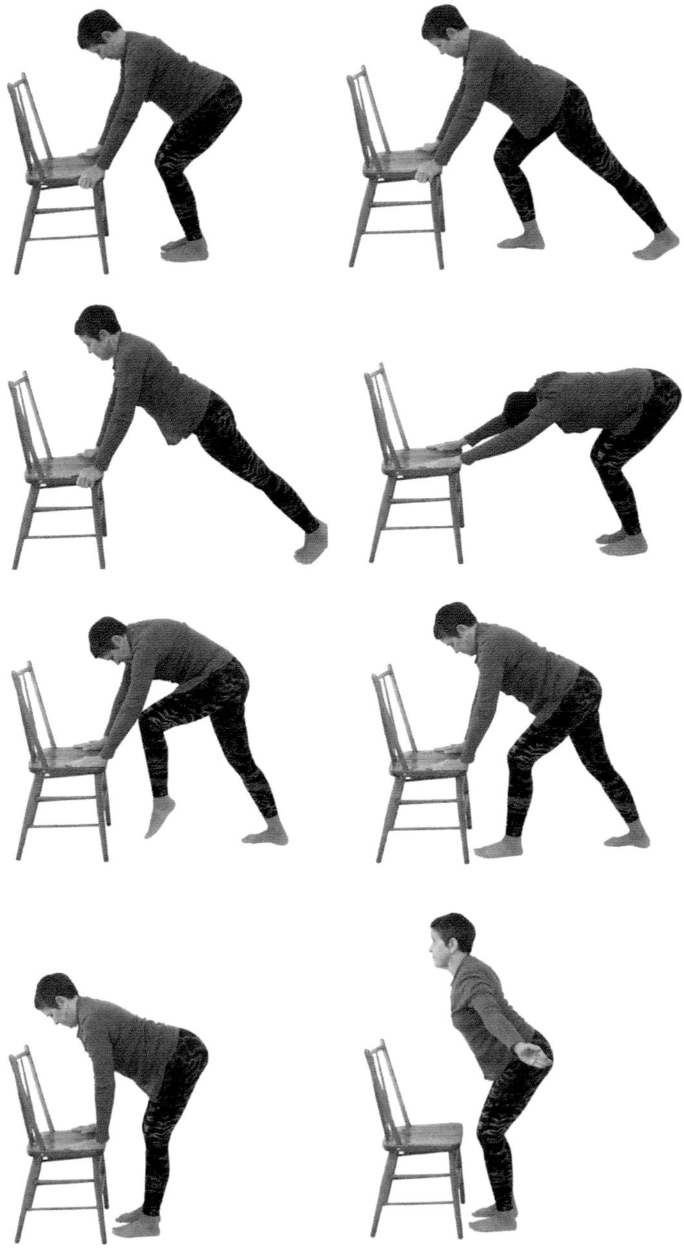

Sun Salutes are requisite in many yoga classes and they often require a lot of Standing Forward Folds. Even if you keep your knees bent during Forward Folds, the spine can still round excessively on both the descent and the rise. Most classes have chairs to lean on, and folding forward to 90 degrees (or with hands propped higher) with knees bent is a safer way to practice with osteoporosis or disc issues. Remember, few yoga teachers object to students choosing safer versions.

Stand a torso's distance from the back of the chair, facing the seat, with your feet about hip-width apart and reasonably parallel at the front of your mat.

Reach your arms out and up, bringing them alongside your ears, with palms facing in. Now widen your arms out to the side again (they'll rotate on the way down) as you bend your knees and fold at hip crease toward the chair, keeping your spine elongated and neutral. Your hands can clasp the outer edges of the chair seat. (Taller people may need to prop the chair seat surface higher with blocks or a folded blanket on a folded sticky mat.)

From there, step your left foot toward the back of your mat, and take a breath. Then step your right foot back to find a chair-supported Plank Pose (if your wrists feel challenged, lift your hips higher). If you are feeling strong here, you can bend your elbows for a *Chaturanga* (Four-Limbed Staff Pose). Hold for 2–3 breaths.

Then, press your hips up and back to find a bent-knee, chair-supported Downward-Facing Dog. You may need to step forward slightly to ground your feet. Let your head move between your upper arms. Stay for 3 breaths.

Next, step your left foot forward, and take a breath. Then step your right foot forward to meet it, returning to your neutral spine Forward Fold.

Rise back up with your knees bent and arms wide.

HALF BIRD DOGS

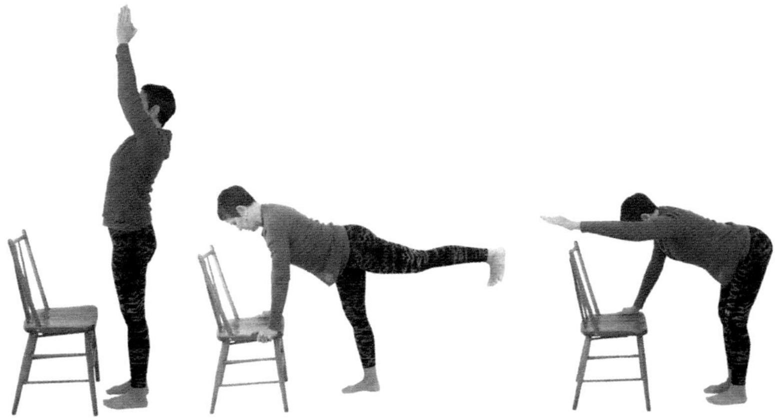

These are effective for strengthening the spinal muscles and building overall core strength.

Stand facing a chair. With your hands clasping the chair's outer edges and your spine neutral, shift your weight onto your right foot and reach your left leg straight back with toes pointing near 90 degrees. Engage your gluteals, both the maximus and the medius, to draw your outer hip inward, and lower your abdomen for support. After 3 breaths, lower your left foot back to the floor and switch sides.

Then, from the same starting position (which you can think of as a "Standing Table Pose"), take your left arm straight out and to the side, palm down. Gradually take your arm up in line with your ear (your palm facing in toward you), keeping your chest level to the floor. As you do this, lightly engage your upper abdominals to support this movement and to avoid shrugging up the shoulder to bring the arm forward. Stay a challenging but reasonable length of time—3 breaths is good—before bringing the arm back out to the side and then back to your starting position. Then from the Standing Table swing your arm around like an elephant swinging its trunk to release tension. Then repeat on the right side.

PURVOTTANASANA (REVERSE TABLE POSE) ON A CHAIR

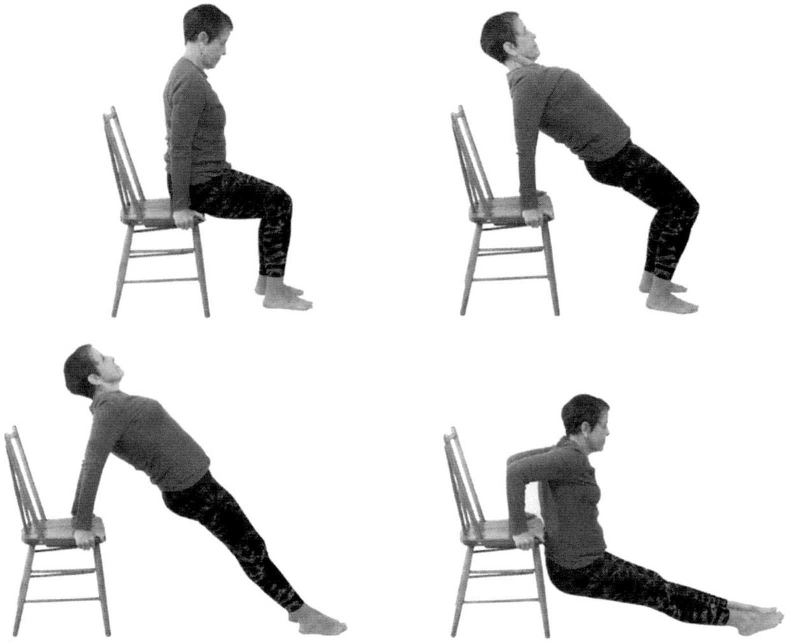

If you have wrist issues, you may need to skip this one or simply sit at the front edge of the chair and reach your hands to the back corners of the chair a few times, opening your chest on the inhalation. These reaches help to counter the forward rolling of the shoulders (kyphosis) and strengthen the arms and shoulders. (This is important because if we should ever have hip or knee surgery or injury we need arm and shoulder strength to help us transfer from a chair to our bed and vice versa during recovery.) You can do one or all three versions depending on how you're feeling.

Version 1

Sit up tall on an armless chair and hold onto the outer edges of the seat. Step your feet away until your legs are somewhat bent, your feet parallel. Inhale, lifting your hips up from the chair as you broaden your chest and keep your chin tucked or head level. Take one breath per lift, then exhale as you sit down. Do 3–5 repetitions.

Version 2

For this version, straighten your legs, with your toes reaching toward the floor. As in the previous version, on an inhalation, lift your pelvis and broaden your chest, keeping your head level and resisting dropping it back. On an exhalation, lower back down. Do 3–5 repetitions of this version as well.

Version 3

This is the same as the previous version, but after you lift up, hold at the top, your head level or your chin a bit tucked. On an exhalation, bend your elbows behind you, dropping your hips slightly below chair level on the way down. On an inhalation, press back up to the open chest position. Try 3–5 repetitions. Don't overdo this exercise or try to dip too low!

VASISTHASANA (SIDE PLANK)

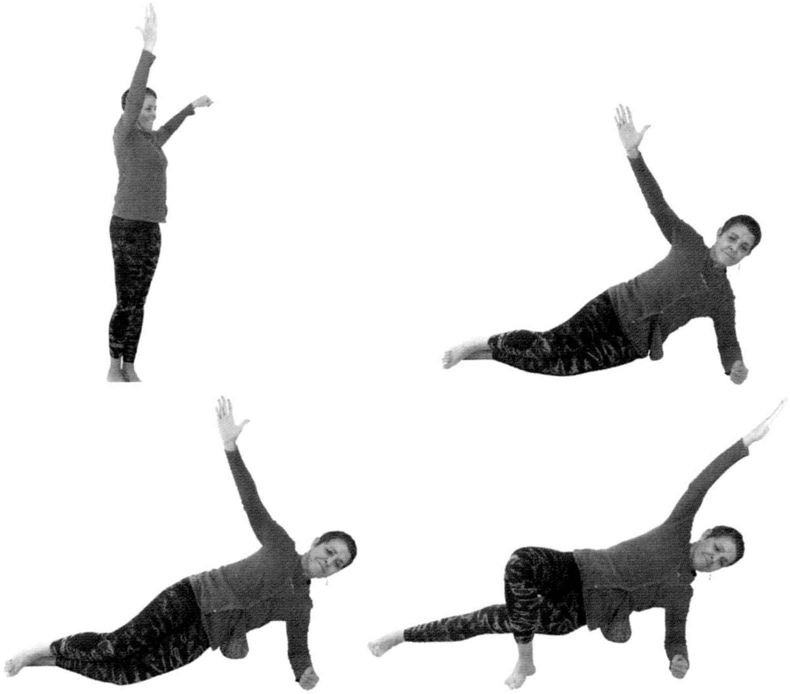

This pose is great for building shoulder strength and balance the curves of the spine. It can be practiced at a wall to avoid too much pressure on the wrist, or on the floor.

To do the pose at the wall, place one hand or forearm on the wall and step your feet out away from the wall so there is modest weight-bearing in the shoulder. Your head will stay in line with your spine. Stay 3–5 breaths.

One way to take this pose to the floor is to begin by lying on your left side and pressing your left elbow down directly below your shoulder, your forearm extending forward and your palm down. Your hips may or may not come off the floor If they do, you can stay with your knees stacked, resting on one knee and outer shin or, for more challenge, you can place your right (top) foot on the floor in front of your left (bottom) knee and lift your hips and left shin away from the floor; you'll be resting on the outer edge of your left foot and the sole of your right foot will press down into the floor.

In any of these versions, your top arm can rest on your hip, reach straight up, or extend overhead in line with the top of your ear. You can build up from 3 breaths in the pose.

INVERSION WITH OSTEOPOROSIS

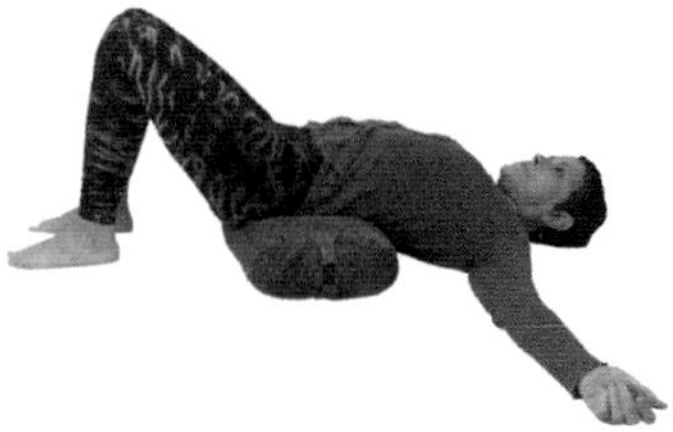

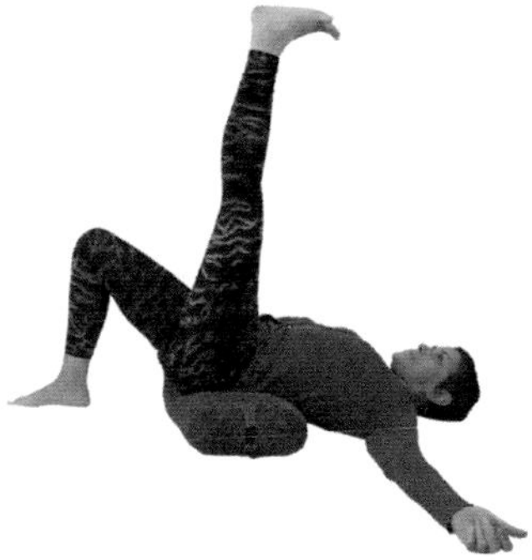

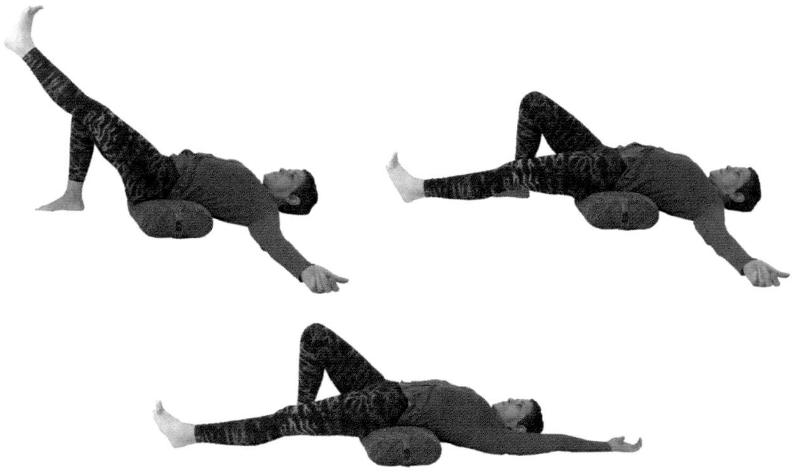

A block may feel like too much pressure on the sacrum in many classes where Supported Bridge and Waterfall (a supported inversion also known as *Viparita Karani*) are taught, especially if that sacral point where the block supports has experienced bone loss. Therefore, a horizontal bolster can be substituted for the block at the sacrum for less pressure on the back. A folded blanket may also feel better for supporting the shoulders and upper back.

Your head rests on the floor. From Supported Bridge supine with your pelvis on the horizontal bolster, take your left heel to the sky and then slowly exhale bringing your left leg forward until your heel almost touches the floor. Do this 3 times, lowering on the exhalation. As you do this, try not to let your pelvis shift to the left side.

Take your left leg back upward to 90 degrees, bring your left heel slowly to the left, controlling the movement by engaging your right transverse abdominal muscles and drawing the left side of your belly to the right side of the belly, to keep the pelvis level. Bring your left leg back to center and slowly lower your heel all the way to the floor. Reach long through your left arm overhead and take 3 deep breaths stretching the left psoas.

Return to your Supported Bridge and do the same on the other side, then stretch both sides together, with your heels on the floor and toes inverted, slightly drawing your tailbone downward and exhaling fully.

SUPPORTED BACKBEND

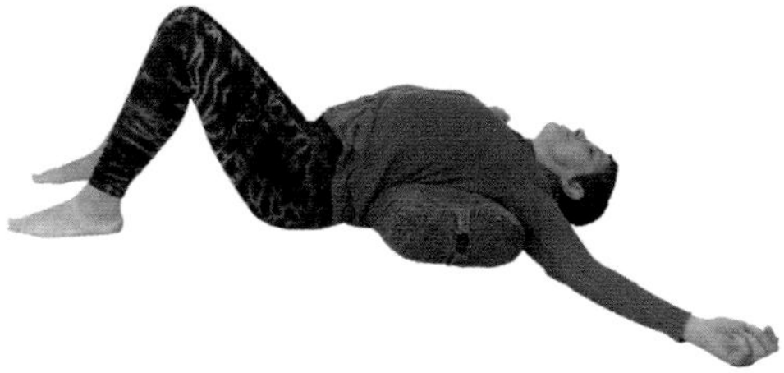

Slither down your bolster until it is beneath your upper back and spread your arms out to a T. Your knees are bent, with your feet on the floor. (Your head may need some support, such as a small pillow or folded blanket if your neck feels over-extended because the bolster is firm and/or tall.) Practice breathing into your abdomen, ribcage, and chest for 5–10 breaths to relieve upper spinal tension.Then, slide the bolster out from under you and roll to a prone position.

DOWNWARD-FACING COBRA

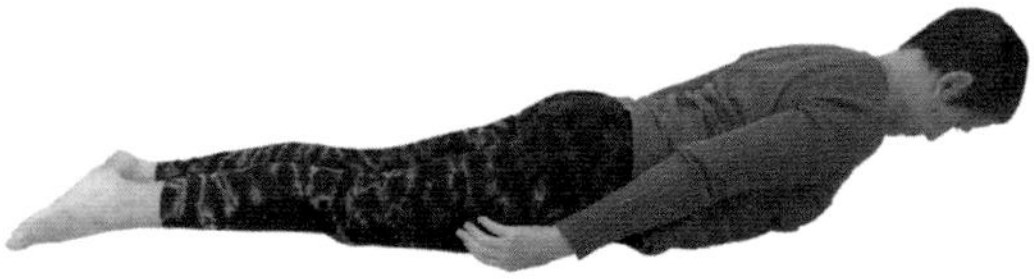

This pose can help to strengthen the back of the neck and help you with finding your optimal head alignment.

Typically, we lift our faces when practicing Cobra Pose, but for this variation, your intention is to keep your chin slightly tucked and to focus on the extension of the upper back (not the neck). Lie on your belly with your inner thighs together, your forehead hovering just above the floor, and your arms resting along your sides with palms facing inward. On an inhalation, keep your gaze down and the back of your neck long as you lift your chest away from the floor. On an exhalation, release. Do 5 lifts and lowers, thinking about lifting the back of your head as you rise.

MAKARASANA (CROCODILE POSE) AND *PARSVA MAKARASANA* (SIDE CROCODILE)

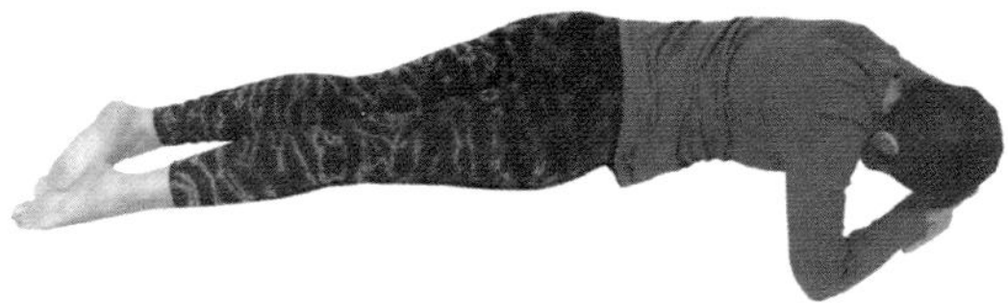

Cross your forearms and rest your forehead on them. Separate your legs as wide as is comfortable for you, allowing your heels to turn in and your toes to turn out if you like. Stay for a few breaths, then come into *Parsva Makarasana* (Side Crocodile), arcing the body to one side by sliding your elbows to the right and then moving your left leg toward your right leg for 5 breaths, then on the other side for 5 resting breaths, with the body in a prone banana shape.

LEGS-ON-A-CHAIR POSE OR OVER A BOLSTER

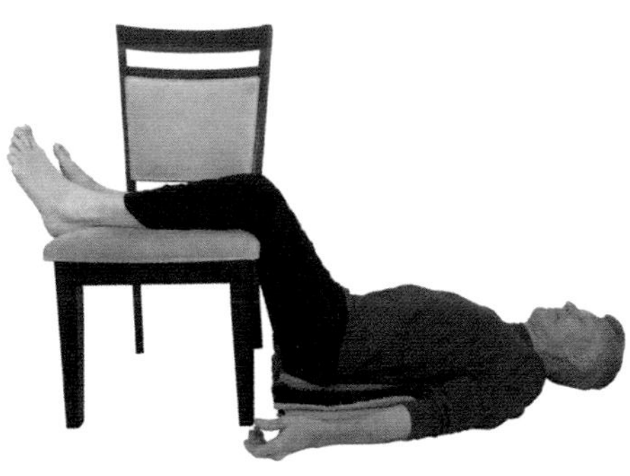

Finish the practice by lying on your back with your calves resting on a chair seat in front of you. You could place a low support (such as a pillow or folded blanket) under your head. If your lower back is uncomfortable against the floor, it may help to place a bolster (horizontally) under your pelvis. Rest here for 5–10 minutes.

There is no need to be afraid of our bodies—we just need to practice smarter! As a Yoga Therapist, it is my intention to help those who are afraid that they can't do yoga (be it following a diagnosis osteoporosis or back injury, stroke, sexual trauma, pregnancy, or something else) to have access to the kind of practice they need. When fear keeps us from exploring this body in which we live, we are missing one of the greatest tools we have for finding wholeness.

CHAPTER 2

Yoga Therapy as Social Activism

The Yoga Therapist can play a powerful role in helping those who are oppressed and disempowered, and in helping people to cope with traumatic incidents in life that may prevent them from helping others in turn. This altruism can be the most impactful part of the healing process. Societal violence and discrimination are often a result of feeling wronged or damaged. Helping to set things right by exemplifying the type of human we'd like to encounter can fortify us when we feel disempowered. We might feel that adding to our already burgeoning plate is more than we can take, but surprisingly, the "giving is receiving" adage frequently proves true.

Often aggression and self-abuse are a result of feeling overburdened, and the thought of adding more to the day, even if it is yoga, may seem daunting. It's important that the Yoga Therapist provides attainable methods—even for *Karma* (service to others) Yoga Therapy—that can be easily understood as simple, practical parts of the day and not as stressful add-ons. Small actions, such as the donation of clothing or helping a neighbor with groceries, are big steps on the path to channeling blocked energy, which can impede feelings of worth.

Empowering the less entitled individual helps us all, as fear underlies societal violence and inequality. A primary motivator of terrorism and war is fear of "the other." But how can Yoga Therapy address societal distrust?

Evolution through Healing Our *Karmas*

In the process of working through the *koshas* (sheaths covering *Atman*), we can come to a realization that we are not our physical bodies (*annamayakosha*), nor are we our emotional states or our tightly held opinions. And every individual has layers through which they must pass toward healing on the soul level. In Yoga Therapy the work is not to direct a person toward their path but more to assist and encourage that person to follow their own course upward and inward.

Patanjali, the eminent scholar of yoga philosophy, laid out a blueprint for our spiritual progression through the integration of the eight limbs of yoga in the *Yoga Sutras*, and Service or *Karma* Yoga is a viable path toward both healing and self-realization.

Patanjali's system begins with an acceptance of virtues and restraints for living our best lives and helping others via the *yamas* and *niyamas*, which are the first two limbs, then moves to *asana*, which is the third limb. According to Patanjali, a primary obstacle for the misalignment of mind and body is imbalance expressed through our physical health. Yoga's movements are designed to help us erase tension deeply enough that we achieve *Savasana* (Corpse Pose). Corpse Pose is often misunderstood. Simply looking dead is not the goal; the goal is to let go of negative attachment to the body and recognize it as a useful layer of existence that does not define us. St. Francis liked to refer to the body as "Brother Ass," saying, "I will ride him, he will not ride me," though I'm certain he took very good care of Brother Ass. Relaxation in *Savasana* is a way of reminding the body who is in charge, and it is very much a learned skill.

Pranayama, which is the fourth limb, and breath practices can lead us to better understand the *pranamayakosha*, our layer of energy.

The release of negative attachment to our physicality brings us to greater sensitivity to how the breath is affecting our mind. Observing the length, balance, tone, and texture of the breath, and the rhythm of our breathing, both in daily seated practice and as we go about our daily lives in the world, helps keep us connected and facilitates better alignment of mind and body.

Fearful breathing is constricted, shallow and high in the chest. You can see the effect of fearful breathing in the muscles of the face, jaw and neck—in states of depression, anxiety or anger, the stress is very frequently visible in the body.

Learning the processes of changing our breathing can have a very positive impact on the underlying emotions. Recent research[1] demonstrates that regulating our breathing can alter hormone levels (cortisol, oxytocin, and vasopressin), thus affecting the stress and relaxation responses that are impacted by these neurohormones.

Patanjali then offers the practice of *pratyahara* (withdrawal of the senses), which is the fifth limb. At this level, a human moves beyond instinctual response and sense memory to more mindfulness-based living. This allows them to better respond to what is happening in the present instead of always basing their judgments on past experience alone.

My daughters recently asked me about how I perceive time. As in: Did their childhoods seem to be a long time ago? It made me think hard about time and instinctual behavior.

To me, my fiercely protective and primal mothering years—the time I spent breastfeeding, noticing their smells of my young children, and being on high alert to keep them from harm—seem to be very recent memories. As do times of grief, such as the deaths of my child, my siblings, and my parents. The sensations are as real now as at the times of the experiences, and it feels as though little time has elapsed. In contrast, the purchase of a car or a move to a new location seem lifetimes ago, even though these events may have happened more recently in my life. It is my sense that very primitive survival instincts keep us bound to memory. I think this applies to all deep life experiences, but it is especially vivid in relation to trauma, often in the form of flashbacks and nightmares.

Post-traumatic stress disorder (PTSD) flashbacks keep an individual in a constant state of stress, as though the traumatic incident they experienced is happening over and over. Our survival requires we remember what hurt us so we don't repeat the behaviors that led to crisis. But those of us who have suffered trauma know that living in constant fear of recurring crisis creates dysfunction, and this dysfunction affects everyone around us. We don't have to forget what's happened, only learn to perceive it as moments in a string of events and that there was time before our traumatic event(s) and after. We'll revisit ways to "unstick" the memory loop in Chapter 7.

Pratyahara begins the process of addressing our primal human fear in the realm of the *manomayakosha* (mind) and works on *vrittis* (latent tendencies). As senses are trained inward, we can more clearly address the source of our fears—sometimes even those that have evolved over lifetimes. The power drained by external grasping is drawn inward for us to use at the level of the mind.

The next rung of yoga is *dharana* (concentration), which is the sixth limb. Here, some (or even all) of the externalization of energy on sense perceptions and fear-based judgments is consolidated in a tangible way in the center of the brain, benefiting the function of the thalamus (which helps us screen out unnecessary or unwanted thoughts) and improving our ability to focus the mind. Many will understand *dharana* as a concentration "on" something, but consider it as a concentration "of" something, as in having more density, potency, and depth. The practice of *prana dharana* places concentrated *prana* at specific locations. This method is asserted by *Pandit* Rajmani Tigunait in his *Living Tantra* series.[2] It also activates the "*pranic* hub" of the hypothalamus and the pituitary and pineal glands. When this area of the brain is activated, often by bringing awareness to the sensation of the breath brushing across the upper part of the nostrils, an awareness of lightness and expansion is felt from the central brain to the temples and it becomes much easier to see oneself as a part of the universe rather than at odds with life. Here, the practitioner can heal the *vijnanamayakosha* and *karmic* issues from past lives. (For techniques for accessing *dharana*, see Chapter 4.)

Dhyana (meditation), which is the seventh limb, is a natural next step in which the concentrated stuff of the mind is brought to rest on an object (e.g., a *mantra*, meditation passage, or the breath) or *bhavana* (intention). Those who try to force the mind to meditate are rarely successful, but consistency and diligence are necessary for nearly all pursuing this path. And when that state of focused peace happens, it's often like falling—no, actually floating—from *dharana* to *dhyana*; there is *ananda* (bliss), and in bliss there is no fear. None. There is a recognition that the universe holds and supports us and there is no "other."

When that state sticks, pure meditation becomes *samadhi*, the result of prolonged, pure meditation, which is the eighth limb. And if being fully present isn't cool enough, the path of *Raja* Yoga (the royal path of meditation) is also a wonderful process that gives meaning and passion to life, regardless of whether we reach permanent enlightenment or not.

The system works, like peeling an onion. Layers of stress, pain, and judgment are peeled away to leave the unadorned truth that we are okay, and that despite all appearances to the contrary, life has our back. Living wholeheartedly becomes less of a challenge.

Yoga Therapy has the capacity to aid the individual in life's journey. It may start with learning therapies for bunions, then surprisingly lead to opening the doors to childhood trauma, and then address a series of distressing life choices. The Yoga Therapist's job is not to take the client back to the origins of their problems (unless they have the appropriate qualifications); but working with movement and breath clearly opens doors that have been stuck and a Yoga Therapist needs to be prepared to listen and use stress management tools to help a client deal with upcoming memories and feelings.

As teachers and therapists we might be tempted to skip the early steps involving the physical and energetic levels of being and simply go right to meditation or mindfulness practices; but recent research by Bessel van der Kolk[3] has shown that following trauma, many people are unable to focus the mind, and that simply sitting can bring flashbacks and related anxiety to the foreground. Reconnection with the sensations in the physical body, however, helps the mind focus.

Do you have to offer a certain set of yoga movements in order to enable a traumatized person to calm down enough for quiet practice? Apparently not. As I mentioned previously, my first teacher would recommend a *mantram* walk for symptoms of trauma, syncing the rhythm of the steps, the breath, and a *mantra.* A friend who worked with communities in Kenya following the post-election violence, in which neighbors committed atrocities toward former friends, found that healing in the community was profoundly aided by Emotional Freedom Technique or "tapping." Children healing from tragedy do well with Play Therapy and Drama or Dance Therapy to help the nervous system recover. So the *asana* level does not have to involve, for example, Warrior Poses or Downward Dogs.

Zen Master Tulku Thondup was fond of saying that the path to healing, self-inquiry, and Self-realization are all the same path, the difference is the point of entry.[4] Each of us has fears and obstacles to overcome in each lifetime, some many more than others. But the journey is the same.

CHAPTER 3

Six Months of Living without Fear

The time of living without fear began about 2 years into recovery from alcohol and prescription drug use, but it certainly wasn't an immediate effect. Though I'd taught *Hatha* Yoga for a number of years and even had a bonafide guru, life had thrown some devastating curves my way, and substance abuse was how I had attempted to cope. This is my story.

The earliest yoga memories I have involve living-room play with my sisters in Springfield, Missouri. Shoulder Stands were "bicycles," and black-footed leotards were the hip thing to wear while you made pretzel shapes with your limbs. It was probably the mid-to-late 60s, and I loved to annoy my family by doing Headstands in Lotus in the back seat of the Dodge Dart. Then came *Lillias, Yoga, and You.* Before PBS came to Springfield, Lillias Folan's show aired on the UHF channel. I grew out my dark hair to match hers, and braided it down one side. Yoga was sooo cool.

As a round, non-athletic girl who hyperventilated during running tests and feared gladiator-style games like dodge ball, yoga was something I could do. Somewhere during those years I remember going to the "Fountain of Health," a "ladies' fitness center," where we jiggled our fat away on belted contraptions and toned our jaw lines with vibrating wands facing a mirror (at 11, I supposed my jaw line was ghastly), encouraged by a goddess of a Swedish woman to sweat and relax our way to her level of perfection. My sister, Elaine—8 years my senior—and I decided to try a yoga class.

The class was led by a charming woman whose school of yoga taught to stretch into approximations of yoga poses and then lie down between each pose in Corpse. We were all advanced in *Savasana* by the end of the series. But this exposure made me hungry for more. Yoga was so cool.

I bought quirky little paperback books with strange poses and bizarre Americanized text about swallowing rags and doing snorting practices. I practiced yoga poses in front of the television during the *Smothers Brothers* and *Dean Martin Show*. I imagined levitating.

I loved the exotic sound of Sanskrit pose names and comically imitated chanting and meditation, maybe feeling a little wicked as the Methodist minister's daughter. Everything about yoga was really cool. It was everything I felt I was not.

At about this same age, 10 or 11, a documentary narrated by poet Rod McKuen caused my life to take a major turn. The show was called *Say Goodbye* and was about the impending extinction of several animal species. There was a graphic scene showing the clubbing of harp seals. "Never," I told my mom, "will I eat an animal again." That "phase" has lasted nearly 50 years and has influenced how I teach and perceive life. Yoga's teachings about the unity of all life were more than cool.

This was my path.

Though I now remember little about what I was leading, I was asked to give yoga lessons to my teen church group. After working with this age group now, as an adult, I imagine there was a good deal of playing around, seeing what we could do and "posturing" (pun intended).

The *Ashtanga* system of yoga was built by Tirumalai Krishnamacharya (considered by many to be the "father" of modern postural yoga) for a group of teenage kids. One of these teens was Patabhi Jois, another was BKS Iyengar. *Asana* at this age channels so much energy for *chakra* development and can play such a key role in brain development that it should be a requirement in high school.

As a teen, I probably needed more practice than most and didn't manage to avoid the pitfalls of depression, eating disorders, and recreational drug use. So much of this could have been avoided by the assistance of a skilled yoga teacher as a guide and mentor. I graduated high school early and started to attend classes at Southwest Missouri State at age 15, planning to be a psychologist one day, or maybe an actress or a famous jazz singer...

During my teens I met my husband, Kevin Richardson, whom I wed in 1979. We married young. Open-minded and freely artistic, the life of vegetarian yogis appealed to our need to grow. We took my National Foundation for the Arts jazz grant money and moved to the San Francisco Bay Area to pursue his graphic arts and my jazz career. We left Springfield right after he graduated from Drury College in the early 80s.

There we had a blessing befall us that shifted our paths forever. We were leading successful lives: I was singing in the best clubs and hotels in the area, and Kevin was breaking ground in the computer graphics mecca of Silicon Valley, yet something was missing. Yes, we had a healthy diet and attended a lot of fitness classes (I taught what was called a "noon stretch" class), but life seemed superficial.

Berkeley bookstores were treasures of Eastern and Western philosophy. I had sung in Unity Churches and was familiar with metaphysics and loved books. My pianist, Buzzy, fed me all I could devour. Theosophy, *Raja* Yoga, *Hatha* Yoga, *Tantra* and *Vedanta* all became fun topics for debate breaks on gigs. We wove in Ramana Maharshi and Ramakrishna with Cannonball Adderly and Bill Evans. Now that's a jam session.

After learning that one of our favorite authors was giving talks in Petaluma, we decided to go see him speak. Hmm, a yogi who didn't do any pretzel poses. He lectured on meditation and its allied disciplines. Eknath Easwaran proceeded to rock our world.

Easwaran's writing was warm and accessible. Kevin and I both came from traditional Christian backgrounds, and he led us to understand the universal truths that underlie all the great schools of thought, including Christianity. Kevin once commented, "I never really understood what Jesus was saying until I heard the Beatitudes explained by a Hindu *brahmin.*" Indeed, Easwaran broached the Christian teachings with the same loving care that he gave the *Upanishads* or the *Dhammapada.*

It was spiritual love at first sight. We came to a Presbyterian church in Petaluma, California expecting to hear a good inspirational writer and speaker, and we watched a lovely 70-year-old man in a tan Nehru jacket sip his tea and tell stories. The audience sat silently, or laughed heartily and enjoyed his lovely flow of verbatim quotes from great teachers and poets interspersed with Sanskrit *shlokas* (a type of sung verse). His stillness ran so deep and his life force was so vibrant that the quality of the light in the sanctuary changed. At the end we sat in meditation with a master. No profound bells or rainbows, just a deep inner calling, telling us this was home.

Kevin and I began hosting *satsang* (spiritual fellowship) at our little place in Albany, California. The groups were small and sincere. Easwaran even came to our house once and our group multiplied tenfold. We would work in Easwaran's *ashram*'s bindery or gardens on weekends and eventually moved near Tomales to be a part of the Blue Mountain Center of Meditation community.

Where was the yoga? Westerners might ask. Easwaran's path was that of a *Jnani*, the path of knowledge. He kept physically active, received regular massages, and was an avid beach walker; however, *asana* was not a part of his regimen. As we progressed, we meditated for up to two hours each morning and evening. Yoga is not about physical postures, though I'll admit that I "cheated" a bit back then and practiced some *asana* to help make meditation more comfortable.

The privilege of studying under an illumined teacher was a rare one. I don't think we fully understood how important it was until we left California to return to Springfield, Missouri. We left because we were expecting our first child, and family was very important to us. The loving support of grandparents was a crucial thread that wove into our understanding of the path.

We bid both the glamour of the West Coast and *ashram* life goodbye and headed into the life of the householder—a true test of the yogi.

When we left our beloved teacher, his words were, "It has been nice knowing you." We truly believed we'd be back, but the intensity of parenthood changes many intentions. We did visit him when our daughter Emily was about three. He called her "the little scholar" due to her love of books and gave her a St. Thérèse medal and a chocolate Santa.

Our *sadhana* (spiritual practice) became childrearing. Two-hour meditations were not easily found and a quick twist to pop the back was sometimes my daily *asana*. I now understand that the *ashram*'s support would have been helpful in these times. A community can offer breaks to needy families, but it's a concept our society knows little of.

I began formally teaching *asana* during this time. My understanding of how this wove into the larger picture of spiritual transformation was limited in the early days, but I loved the practice and studied under many fine teachers, mainly from the Iyengar lineage. I enjoyed the attention to alignment, safety, and accessibility via the use of props that this type of yoga offered, but the anatomically specific, often militaristic, style of teaching was not my voice. When teachers would visit the Midwest, I'd make the trek to encounter the joy of *vinyasa* and alignment in the 90s with Shiva Rea and John Friend; and finding my music in the practice, feeling the energetic dance of yoga was more like my life as a musician and it sang to my heart. Bliss on the mat—that was it! I later came to love the *Kundalini* Yoga practice in the same way, moving subtle energy by not-so-subtle means. All of the differing schools of yoga would eventually affect how I practice Yoga Therapy.

We had some early-stage miscarriages during the time before Emily was born, and my early labor and placental issues with our firstborn should have given us a clue that this parenting process would not be easy. Many years later we found that I had complications in childbirth due to celiac disease (extreme gluten intolerance). With my being anemic and sick a good deal of the time during pregnancy, our second child, Claire, arrived very early weighing 1 pound 11 ounces. She spent three tortured months in neonatal intensive care. We finally brought her home, only to have her fall ill with respiratory problems. What would have been a cold to most children set off her bed alarms and panicked us (we'd seen her go through so much already). When we ran from ER to the doctor's office for days, our pleas were ignored by hospital staff. She rapidly became so sick that she was placed back on a respirator, but it was the wrong caliber—an error, we were told, many doctors might have made. When she was airlifted to a children's hospital in Arkansas, her lungs were irreparably damaged. Her big sister Emily, Kevin, and I said goodbye to her a few days later.

Our faith was shaken at its roots. Easwaran contacted us during this time to let us know he had helped her make her transition and was there for us now. This was one of our only consolations.

One year later we gave birth to beautiful twin girls, and grief took a back seat.

PTSD, however, did not take a back seat, as the disconnect from my physical body and my zombie-like functioning should have indicated. Interestingly, my mother had been severely abused as a child and suffered from trauma (and celiac disease), and as an adult, she was often overmedicated. Recent research on the children of holocaust survivors shows that even the next generation of those who experience trauma have lower-than-normal cortisol levels and are less able to resist the effects of PTSD. It was certainly so with me.[1]

I loved my girls with what sanity I had left and felt fiercely protective (probably hypervigilant) about all three of them. My dreams and daytime thoughts compelled me to worry endlessly about their survival. My oldest would go to visit fellow homeschoolers and I had thoughts that she would never come home. I checked my babies to make sure they were breathing multiple times during naps and at night. I resisted letting even their grandparents hold or care for the little ones and insisted that Emily wash her hands far too often. To say I was in a constant state of suspense is an understatement. My anxiety was off the scale.

One often looks back on life and sees pivotal moments that open doors and offering them to the public after the fact is sometimes a blessing and a curse that risks revealing too much. Coming to terms with addiction is one of those pivotal points.

After our heartbreaking loss and then the complete surprise of twins just one year later, grief was shoved under a rug of non-stop activity: caring for children, Kevin working three jobs, homeschooling, teaching yoga, and singing in Kansas City. We were the running wounded.

An old *samskara* (an addictive mental scar that emerges again and again through the course of one's life) came to the fore. As a performer, I had always had the tendency to drink, and this became a place to hide. Over the years a *samskara* worsens when we stop doing something for a while but then pick it back up again. Neural connections become stronger and the mind seeks the effect of the addictive substance. The numbing sickness, the injuries, the shakes, the dull, yellow-framed eyes were not a part of the yogic lifestyle. You might ask, "Didn't yoga help?" Of course it did! But *asana* is not a panacea, and in times of dark PTSD, meditation can simply seem an empty activity. Plus with nighttime nursing and children up all hours of the day, meditation became a little attempt at focus while holding one or two babies with a little spiritual reading in the rocking chair.

Our oldest daughter watched her parents emotionally deteriorate, and the old drinking habit from my days as a club singer returned and took priority.

Several drastic attempts at recovery and hospitalization in psychiatric wards failed until, one day, I sat in my car in the early morning, with my purchase of wine, ready to begin the daily blur. I thought of my spiritual teacher and the noble goals he had instilled in us to make the world better. He seemed far away, and I began talking aloud to Easwaran in my car. "What happened? Can you help me now?" Easwaran had passed a couple of years prior, and I felt a little foolish talking to my deceased teacher. Then two days later, two books came in the mail from the Blue Mountain Center of Meditation. I had not ordered them, but they were addressed to only me, while all other orders we had placed were addressed to both Kevin and me. These books were the updated edition of Easwaran's classic *Passage Meditation*, and the most beautiful passages of verse and prayer ever assembled, *Timeless Wisdom*, which Easwaran recommended for meditation (as a former literature professor his taste and translation were elegant). I took it that Easwaran was telling me to start at the beginning and relearn meditation and his dynamic eight-point program as if they were new to me, and I did. In acceptance of sobriety as part of my spiritual journey, I was led to a simple, well-run outpatient program, which helped reinstate my will to live. And that living began with hot intensity. My children's existence became so clear and sweet that I forgot about risks of loss and enjoyed each moment. I slept little during this time, only needing four hours a night, practiced *asana* morning and evening, and spent several hours each day in meditation.

My diet was sparse and *sattwic* (simple and full of life force). I walked and repeated Easwaran's mantra "*Hare Rama Hare Rama Rama Rama Hare Hare, Hare Krishna, Hare Krishna Krishna Krishna Hare Hare.*" Clarity began to return and at that time I was introduced to *tantric* breathing practices by a visiting *Pandit*, a man esteemed for his wisdom or learning. Coincidentally, he had known Easwaran and said that Easwaran was a man who lived every word he taught. I wanted to embody that as well and live what Easwaran taught and teach it myself.

The *tantric* breathing techniques tripped the switch, as though there was a change in my brain chemistry on a very deep level. I experienced many of the classical effects of *kundalini* rising, both in meditation and sometimes waking from sleep in an ecstatic state of near giddiness. A massage therapist was overwhelmed by the vibration of my spine and brain, and my husband would feel the often intense vibration from his side of the bed. "Like magic fingers!" he would say (in reference to those coin-operated jiggly massaging beds from the 60s). My voice, skin, body odor, and eyes changed during this time and students were drawn to classes from long distances. I'd laugh when they called me "teacher" or "*guru.*" I just felt clear for the first time. I'd alter my focus slightly and my friends or pets would no longer be solid. Plant, animal, and human life was dynamic and fused; I'd see life as almost molecular, and the interaction of all things made perfect sense. Long passages of text or scripture I had read would come up from my memory and I could summon them as if from nowhere; answers to difficult questions were granted without stress.

Life itself became *sadhana*. Who I was before dissolved, and injuries to those around me began to heal. The seeds of practice began to grow, and I learned that *samskara* thrown into the fire of life force brings such abiding joy that no lure could draw me back. The intensity of life became vibrant.

I have heard it said that those who thirst most for wine thirst most for the waters of life, an accurate assessment of addictive tendency. When applied negatively, that thirst manifests as addiction but when it is applied positively, as in music, learning, yoga, or service to those who need help, there is always a passion for more. That is what I felt: a passion for more.

A favorite meditation passage of mine during that time was from the *Rig Veda*: "Release me from my sorrows which hold me as ropes hold a calf, I can not even open my eyes without the power of your love."[2] By the grace of my teacher, Easwaran, the ropes fell away and life became far from ascetic or deprived. I had freedom in the world, not from the world.

Students have accused me of being a hardliner on social and ethical discipline, especially during training. My path has been one of very strong addiction, and the more difficulty we have overcoming selfish attachment, the more *prana* (spiritual force) it has behind it. Power is power, and can be funneled upward or downward, meaning one can take an electrical current and cause brain damage or use the same current to save a life. The same is true of the power behind addiction. We lose ourselves or we perhaps find out who we are for the very first time, depending on which direction we take. As noted yoga teacher and recovery expert Tommy Rosen often says, "Recovery from addiction is recovery of the Self."[3] Conversely, for people to give up the wealth of sharing simple joys, a late night chat with an old friend, a chocolate truffle with the family, or a glass of wine to toast a wedding would be an obstruction to living fully. We were given human bodies to love and taste the wonders of being alive. The balance is living in beauty, totally free of attachment. As for me, I'll toast with cider and dance!

Doors began opening toward the late 90s, and it seemed the right thing to open a yoga teacher training center and pursue my own studies in yoga therapeutics.

I had been reticent to share the deeper teachings of yoga in the classes I offered due to fear of alienating students, but Easwaran's intervention in my life gave me confidence to bring his translations of the *Bhagavad Gita*, the *Upanishads*, the *Dhammapada*, and classics of Christian mysticism into what was often considered a fitness atmosphere. Some students opted out, wanting only physical practice, while others were intrigued or had been searching for more in their yoga practice. The ancient texts that sang to my spirit were a joy to many. We learned together how to clear the temple of the body on the mat to make it a fit home for the *Atman*, the soul.This ideal has infused my Yoga Therapy practice as well, though I keep sessions pretty clinical and want people to have their own "ah-ha" moments.

I don't take time often enough to remember what a blessing it is to have such a direct weave of my work and my *sadhana*. Teaching yoga and Yoga Therapy demands that I study, meditate, have a strong personal practice, and continue to learn.

I'd like to add a bit more to the story of the pivotal point for me. Even though Easwaran's path and methodology were quite different, I have no doubt he led me to *Pandit* Rajmani Tigunait, spiritual head of the Himalayan Institute. I had studied with *Tantric* Yoga teacher Rod Stryker, founder of Parayoga, on a few occasions and had enjoyed his strong *asana* and unique use of breath in the practice. He introduced me to *tantric kriyas* (actions done with specific intention) and spoke of his teacher, *Pandit* Tigunait. He mentioned his teacher was coming to St. Louis in 2009. I went to meet *Pandit* Tigunait on his Living *Tantra* Tour.

Tantra is an ancient school (not a religion) that teaches us to weave all the elements of our lives into the sacred. All we do is part of paring away all that is not the truth of our being. Every choice we make, all day long, is a step on the path. We don't run from life, we immerse ourselves wholly in life. All experience is grist for the mill and consequently nourishment for the soul. The Western take on *Tantra* is often to make the profane or vulgar sacred by emphasizing orgies or drunkenness; on the contrary, in a traditional *tantric* practice we weave the threads we most cherish into our tapestry. Those threads which no longer serve us are left behind without attachment.

The day I left to attend the Panditji's (a term of endearment from his students) workshop I picked up Easwaran's *Words to Live By* for the month of May and read this quote from Ramana Maharshi: "If you go on working with the light available, you will meet your master, as he himself will be seeking you."[4] Easwaran's commentary goes on to define a *guru* as "one who is so heavy that he or she cannot be shaken."

Meeting *Pandit* Tigunait was just what I needed after months of intense practice and refocused energy. His scholarly wisdom sprang from a seemingly endless well of study with his teacher *Swami* Rama of the Himalayas. He tends to dance about subject matter and you don't even know what you learned sometimes until later, like a gardener planting seeds of needed information.

I had the opportunity to speak to him at break from the lecture in St. Louis and asked him if he knew Easwaran. Indeed he did, and he loved and respected him dearly. While on break between lectures, Panditji took quite a bit of time to answer some of my personal questions regarding Easwaran. He called me to the platform the next day to tell me a story about congratulating Easwaran on his translation of the *Bhagavad Gita.* He told of how he had asked Easwaran for his favorite verse, then Panditji, so like Easwaran, sang the passage from the scripture called the "Illumined Man," which was both Easwaran's and Gandhi's favorite verse. I felt such joy and gratitude. I was home again! Other amazing things happened that weekend, like finding a tiny statue of Kali totally buried under wood chips in a Catholic meditation labyrinth after Panditji had spoken about the deity. But the most wonderful things were the teachings he offered, which deepened my practice profoundly and immediately—teachings I could bring home to share with my students and which they in turn could teach to others, especially the transformative practice of *Prana Dharana,* which I will cover in detail in Chapter 4.

Later, I went to a follow-up workshop with Sandra Anderson, a long-time student of *Swami* Rama and *Pandit* Tigunait, and met a wise mentor. On arriving at Sandy's workshop my friend Christine told me that Panditji had called her home that morning to send me a welcome. I was puzzled but pleased. Why a welcome to me? Later that day, Sandy consented to come to my studio in a few months to offer more of the deep teachings of *Tantra*. Before she came to Springfield, I visited the Himalayan Institute and spoke with friends and *Pandit* Tigunait. He jumped right into global issues in our private talk, expressing a sense of urgency about our Earth. My question for him was, "What can we do to help your work?" He knew immediately of my school's outreach to underserved areas of the community and told me we were very much on track and that those living in fear, shame, and trauma deeply needed the teachings. I went home with a heart full of intentions to reshape my corner of the world, marveling at my good fortune in life.

As dramatic as some of these events were, the most memorable was this state of fearlessness. I had always had anxiety about driving, worried endlessly about my children, panicked when speaking before groups, and often stressed about what people were thinking. Now all of that was gone! I saw everything as logical and in order, a tangible protective bubble was in place and my reaction in apparently negative situations was "What can I do to make this better? How can I be of help?", whereas before I would have looked for someone to whom I could lament, because I feared making a wrong move. My behavior may have looked like insanity from the outside, or ego, or desire for success or notoriety. At the time I didn't care how it looked—for 6 months, having turned over the keys, I was almost unbearably happy.

But what happened to that state after those 6 months? Why wasn't I able to maintain this heightened state of awareness? In a word, negativity, and more deeply, fear, got in the way. They took me back down. I was directing a Non-Profit 501(c)3 yoga education center. We trained and certified yoga teachers to work in underserved areas of the community, drug and alcohol recovery, early childhood development and senior centers, schools, a branch of juvenile detention, English as a Second Language (ESL) classes, cancer centers, developmental disability programs, and more. A part of the teacher training was supervised instruction in an area of passion for the student in training. For instance, if they had family members with multiple sclerosis (MS), perhaps they would do their research and practice in that area; or if they wanted to work with kids in Headstart Centers, we'd try to arrange opportunities to teach there alongside me or a senior student teacher. We offered scholarships to help those who couldn't afford the cost of a 500-hour teacher training and sliding scale public classes. My board of directors was initially enthusiastic about our thriving course of good works, but gradually their enthusiasm waned, as the budget was barely balanced and donations for a humanitarian yoga center were not something the public yet understood. Fear of failure took over the venture and to my dismay our hard-earned non-profit status dissolved. The board insisted my family had to earn more money than we were for running an education center, even though it seemed that we always miraculously had "loaves and fishes" aplenty. Along with the transition from non-profit to for-profit came criticism and jealousy from the previously supportive yoga community. I may have appeared to be an egomaniac, looking for fame through humanitarian efforts. Petty rumors began about the yoga center and our supposed ulterior motives. There was jealousy since we were now competing in the yoga market. I finally cracked; it got to me. Fear and negativity gnawed at my good intentions and new-found reality.

The book *Kundalini Tantra* speaks about losing a level of *samadhi* as "falling from the heart," and that is how this felt. It also says that it is very hard to return once it happens. That has been my experience.

While I can still enter into a deep meditation and feel tangible connection with higher energy, and have times of insight that I can't explain, there is still fear, still doubt, in my daily life. The intense discipline is more complicated in an older body, I intend to relocate the discipline via seated practice and breath work, because life doesn't last forever and fearlessness is worth any effort.

As a big step in our spiritual journey, in 2015 our twins graduated high school and were accepted to NYU film school, so Kevin and I sold our home and nearly everything we owned and moved to the Himalayan Institute in Pennsylvania, not far from New York City, to continue study. I was privileged to provide Yoga Therapy at their clinic, and often in *Ayurvedic* retreats, with many clients from all over the world. We now live near the Institute and I create article and video content for *Yoga International*, which is an affiliated platform.

My opportunities to study Yoga Therapy from so many noble lineages is a gift I don't take lightly; and in this process I see yoga transforming lives in ways no one would have believed back in the early misunderstood days of yoga in the USA. Being able to witness (and participate in) the fusion of ancient and modern teachings is something I've longed to see. And now, constantly coming across new scientific research that validates what I'm teaching makes Yoga Therapy a very exciting place to be.

These words from Hafiz of Shiraz speak to me when facing challenging and frightening times: "I wish I could show you when you are lonely or in darkness the astonishing light of your own being."[5] Even though I don't always feel invincible, I know that the underlying truth is that we are in fact the astonishing light and that light can be trusted.

One of the largest contributing factors in the shift from waking up fearful and living with a sense of support is *tapas* (discipline). Some translations of the word associate *tapas* with heat, the burning of old patterns in the sacrificial fire. *Tapas* takes precedence over, and burns, old daily patterns.

Discipline does not mean leading a deprived, dull life, though. *Tapas* is, instead, a way of trading mundane pleasure for joy. Many people find that this trade-off imbues them with the fearlessness they are looking for. It's as though the purpose of a higher calling opens gates of courage, allowing them to do what had previously seemed terrifying.

I find that it is often difficult to persuade my clients that their favorite old patterns may not be helping them on their journey to wellness and joy—that these habits may, in fact, glue them to fearful living. The Yoga Therapist/teacher can only offer suggestions and be a personal example; it is up to the individual to apply the new lifestyle patterns to their day (and, in truth, many people come to Yoga Therapy strictly for physical benefits and have no interest in yoga's deeper offerings or the limbs beyond *asana*).

For those who choose to weave yogic lifestyle practices into their daily tapestry, markers appear.

Choice as a Therapeutic Tool

When a garden-fresh sweet potato sounds better than New York cheesecake.

When the day-long dullness of sleeping two hours longer and skipping meditation feels more like a punishment than a treat.

When we decide to go to the park and enjoy nature instead of staying home and bingeing on Netflix.

These are all good signs that our yoga practices are hitting their mark and moving beyond the mat to changing our habits and behaviors.

Yet even yoga practitioners face those moments when we know that third glass of wine or second dessert will likely lead to regret, but we still find ourselves taken in by indulgences and the fleeting pleasure of the out-of-control moment. It's an age-old quandary.

When we understand that with ability comes responsibility, we're able to realize that the human mind has the capacity to not only say "no" to cravings but to completely enjoy the higher alternative.

As we discussed earlier, the word *tapas* can be translated as discipline or austerity. Some translators liken it to penance, suffering, pious activity, or misery. It certainly doesn't sound like there is much happiness to be found in that! But the sages spoke of the joy of self-discipline, the sweetness of sweat and service, and the movement of *tapas* to *tejas* (pure radiance). It is one of the basic tenets of yogic living. We deal every moment with the "I want" versus "I need" dilemma, and some teachers tell us that making the higher choices is what differentiates humans from animals (though I have known some highly altruistic animals!). When we understand that with ability comes responsibility, we're able to realize that the human mind has the capacity to not only say "no" to cravings but to completely enjoy the higher alternative.

But while discipline can be fruitful (and even delightful!), excess in austerity can result in addiction of another type, especially when we fixate on personal appearance or ego-based attainments. The Buddha referred to the middle path: not reckless behavior on Saturday night and starving the rest of the week, but consistent, pleasant ease in behavior.

Easwaran[6] often told this story, and it was recounted in a *Yoga International* article:

> I can give one small example of this at my own expense. South India is full of cashew trees, and when I was a boy, the path to school led through a cashew nut orchard. Everyone likes cashew nuts, and the tree in fruit is an artist's delight—beautiful colors made to captivate the eye. So a cashew orchard is a double temptation, and we boys, transparently honest on other occasions, regularly stopped to rob those particular trees on our way to school.
>
> I must have done this throughout my career in high school. Then, after India's independence, all our cashews began to be exported to the United States of America—a matter of foreign exchange—and those delicious nuts disappeared from my life. For the rest of my time in India, I got no nearer to a cashew than the factories where they were processed.
>
> I thought I had forgotten this childhood passion until many years later in the U.S., when a hospitable friend with whom I was staying discovered this skeleton in my cupboard. She brought a big tin of cashew nuts and left it on my table as a surprise.
>
> That evening I was reading the Gita with deep concentration when I suddenly discovered that my right

hand was missing. I set the book aside and looked for it. It was hidden in the cashew tin!

I was utterly astonished. My mind and I are on fairly good terms, so I said sternly, "You can't be doing what I think you are doing! Nibbling without my approval?" My mind looked sheepish. "Boss, you don't think I would do that, do you? I was only trying to find out what was in the tin."

Clearly, this was time to nip a compulsive attachment in the bud before it got out of hand.

I did not eat a single cashew that day, though my mind was craving for them. All those old, fierce memories were aroused, but every time they clamored for cashews, I went for a fast walk repeating my mantram or gave my mind something spiritual to read instead.

The next day was the same, and the next. For a few days, I read with my book supported by both hands.

Finally the craving went away. I forgot about cashew nuts completely. That day I told my mind, "Now you can take a handful and enjoy."

This is freedom. And, let me tell you, cashew nuts eaten in freedom taste a hundred times better than nuts eaten under the tyranny of a craving.

He didn't throw them away; he grew his own character through *tapas* and then enjoyed both his cashews and his discipline. Easwaran told us often that we all have that capacity.

Discipline is not punishment; it's freedom of choice. Those cravings own us; shaking them loose is an unburdening. We no longer fear losing the desired substance or state.

Sometimes setting up a "payment plan" for ourselves—like fasting only one day a week for clarity or empathy (not weight loss) and then donating the money saved to a passionate cause—is the middle path. It's not so much eating the sugar-free alternative cheesecake as it is learning to savor the well-prepared kale served by and enjoyed with a loved one. Easwaran also often spoke of going out with friends, especially children, for treats. This is very different from a pint of Ben and Jerry's on the sly. Enjoying the faces, the voices, the experience of family and friends, and eating a small helping of celebratory ice cream with attention and not self-indulgence is a beautiful tightwire of *tapas*, which brings joy—real joy. Discipline is not punishment; it's freedom. The fruits of *tapas* are what fuel our development, allowing us to give our best to life.

With this freedom comes fearlessness and a greater understanding of the distinction between what is pleasurable and that which benefits all. The *Katha Upanishad* aptly illustrates and defines the difference.

> "There is nothing else that I want, O Death, and I can have no better teacher than you. I am your devoted disciple; give me instruction." Pleased, the King of Death begins. "Nachiketa," he says, "as a human being, you have been born with the capacity to make choices. No other creature has this capacity, and no human being can avoid this responsibility. Every moment, whether you see it or not, you have a choice of two alternatives in what you do, say, and think."[7]

As Eknath Easwaran discusses in his translation, *Essence of the Upanishads* (particularly this portion quoted from the *Katha Upanishad*), these alternatives have precise, Sanskrit names that have no English equivalent: *preya* and *shreya*:

> Preya is what is pleasant. Shreya, what is beneficial. Preya is that which pleases us, that which tickles the ego. Shreya, on the other hand, has no reference to pleasing or displeasing. It simply means what benefits us—that which improves our health or contributes to our peace of mind.[8]

And from the translation of the *Katha Upanishad* by *Pandit* Tigunait:

> The good (shreya) and the pleasant (preya) are two different things. They motivate a person to pursue two different goals. The one who embraces the good meets with auspiciousness. But the one who embraces the pleasant is lost.[9]

This isn't always a concept that gets a lot of applause. In fact, it may even be ridiculed:

> "You're having fruit for dessert? Come on, there are cookies. Diet, *shmiet*, you only live once!"
>
> "Getting to bed by 10:00? Your mommy must be very proud."
>
> "Get a sitter. This will be a fun, grown-up evening out. Your kids will understand missing the camping trip!"

Many Sanskrit words have interesting pairings and are considered opposites. *Preya* and *shreya* are similar to *rama* (often translated as the source of joy), and *kama* (the pursuit of pleasure). An Indian saying goes, "When crossing the rickety rope bridge one whispers, 'Rama, Rama, Rama,' calling the name of the Lord for protection. When reaching safety, it's '*kama, kama, kama.*'" So, it's back to business as usual and the pursuit of what appeals to us. Is there something wrong with pursuing pleasure? No, we are entitled to the human experience in its fullest. But what does that mean?

I seriously doubt Mick Jagger had been reading the yogic scriptures when he and Keith Richards wrote that you can't always get what you want, but if you try you might find what you need. It's true though. What we need is what is beneficial. It's why we have this little Jiminy Cricket of a conscience on our shoulder whispering that someone else may need that last pancake. The difference between what we want and what we need seems to be the baseline criterion for the spiritual path.

In his inspirational talks, Easwaran would often liken *preya* to a handsome, mustached, hairy-chested salesman who can talk us into purchasing the goods every time, while timid *shreya* is like the classic librarian with her hair in a prim updo, until you take time to notice her. And then she shakes down her hair and her deep, clear eyes come out from behind the thick glasses. Beauty or flash? What do we want? Or more importantly, what do we need?

But we want evidence, right? And we ask, "What's in this for me in the long run?" I'm not a big fan of laboratory animal studies, but my good friend and colleague in teacher trainings, Dr. Scott Zimmerman, does Alzheimer's research. He cites one study done with mice in two environments:[10] One habitat had food and a wheel to run on. The other was a mouse playground—food, mirrors, other mouse buddies, tubes, and materials for nesting fun. Guess which mice did not succumb to Alzheimer's as readily? Nope, the wheel-and-cage group. Less distraction, more exercise, more benefit. Mice run ridiculous distances in the wild. It's what they do naturally, scavenging and seeking. Less distraction and less pleasure added up to more time to do what mice need.

Scott's own research at Missouri State University found another interesting piece of the Alzheimer's puzzle.[11] When he and his group of researchers looked at forced exercise (treadmill running) compared with voluntary exercise (wheel running), they found that, while both delayed Alzheimer's disease, voluntary provided more benefit than forced. So, choosing to do what's beneficial, like exercise, provides more benefit than being forced to do what is beneficial. This points to the efficacy of doing what is right for the joy of feeling better. If we exercise because of a societal weight standard or because we are made to feel fearful, guilty, and pressured, we may lose weight or gain some muscle mass, but the benefits may not hold unless our hearts are behind the change. On the other hand, freely making healthy choices, because we recognize both their long-term value and the present joy that they bring, rearranges our old habit patterns (*samskaras*) and draws us toward *shreya* patterns.

Have you ever been the one who spends time playing with the kids at the barbecue rather than indulging in beer-driven adult conversation? Who takes your day off to build homes for low-income families? Who gives your energy and vacation time to help communities stricken by disaster? Who chooses meditation time over Facebook time? Then you have likely experienced the lowering of stress and ensuing happiness that occurs with selflessness and service. In fact, the same stress hormones that are lowered by dark chocolate are impacted by our own acts of kindness!

But this brings up a question that arose in a *Bhagavad Gita* class that I recently attended, with one of my favorite teachers,

Dr. Rolf Sovik, President and Spiritual Director of the Himalayan Institute, as well as a clinical psychologist, writer and *Pandit.* The inquiry was, "Isn't craving higher consciousness a selfish craving?" Following the question, Dr. Sovik asked the group to identify the nature of craving, and a series of unpleasant words came up: greed, ego, selfishness, indulgence, even avoidance of fear. Dr. Sovik agreed that those words were fitting, but noted that there was an important one that we'd left out: impermanence. This is often the actual impetus for our less-than-stellar choices and behaviors. We choose what is appealing for now, while ignoring hints, visions, or nigglings from the conscience about negative long-term impact. Yet, when our desires and cravings (and the power they possess to direct our course) are funneled instead into the lasting, permanent good of the soul, then we are operating from *shreya.* Making effort to grow spiritually is never time wasted. As the *Bhagavad Gita* (2:40) tells us, "On this path, effort never goes to waste, and there is no failure. Even a little effort toward spiritual awareness will protect you from the greatest fear."[12] And this is true even when we feel like we are just treading water.

So, it may not feel like joy right now, but measuring our efforts on the joy/pleasure scale is something we can do to keep the good flowing.

CHAPTER 4

Being Okay with Not Being Okay

The Roles of Meditation and the Breath

In his book *Buddha's Brain* Rick Hanson says:

> If I know one thing for sure, it's that you can do small things inside your mind that will lead to big changes in your brain and your experience of living... You really can nudge your whole being in a better direction every day.
>
> When you change your brain, you change your life.[1]

I have spent years at odds with the idea that thinking about things getting better will actually effect the changes you want to see. For many years I worked in New Age churches that encouraged speaking only positive words and envisioning the car or house you wanted to manifest. It appeared to work for some, but for others, there was still cancer and job loss, and then I lost my child in spite of hundreds of people sending prayers and affirmations. I decided at that time it doesn't work. You can't prevent the wheels of *karma* from turning and make life an ever-triumphant saga.

My perspective on rewiring the brain for a better life has shifted more recently. A few weeks ago I read a social media discussion about Thich Nhat Hanh's famous meditation: "Breathing in I calm my body, Breathing out I smile, Dwelling in the present moment, I know this is a wonderful moment."[2] The question was raised, "What if it isn't a wonderful moment? What if you have chronic illness, are being abused, or have a beloved parent on their deathbed?" And I definitely relate to that question.

Our family has had the ascending bubble pop and have been free-falling for months with one daughter's chronic Lyme disease out of remission (putting her in need of care and support), serious financial hardship, resurgence of addictive patterns, my advanced osteoporosis, and seemingly insurmountable student debt—concerns that took our breath away and left us smile-less. "Knowing this is a wonderful moment" seemed anything but the truth.

But the turmoil of the human condition isn't the "present moment" that Hanh is talking about. He is referring to that change of brain state that Rick Hanson refers to: that going within and experiencing the broadness at the temples or sensation of inner light that we've trained the mind to find in interior practice.

Animals can give us an understanding of being okay when things aren't okay. As I was walking home by the river yesterday, I saw a young deer, just old enough to be past the dappled haunches stage. She was nibbling something green at the roadside and didn't care that I was passing. She even gamboled about playfully and went back to her verdant snacking. A few yards away there was a palm-sized bunny doing the same thing—munching fervently on a stalk, then frisking about in the "wonderful moment." Then a car came by and both animals went undercover. I thought about the lifespan of such creatures and that the odds for them making it to maturity are probably not that good; they have little defense against predators and vehicles. Yet, here they were eating what they needed, being on their own, living the life they came here to live, and for a moment things were perfect. That's the lesson.

Brené Brown talks a good deal about the value of accepting one's vulnerability for self-transformation and how it is a big part of healing.[3] Pema Chödrön, in her book *When Things Fall Apart*, recommends moving toward pain rather than away.[4] In some ways, it reminds me of the child digging in the manure, just knowing there has to be a pony in there somewhere. Facing the facts that life will be difficult and that we, like my woodland friends, function best when we stay real and vulnerable helps keep us from being overcome by anxiety, fear, and pain (and from getting hit by cars).

There is a *tantric* practice called *Prana Dharana* that transforms the ability of the mind to focus and has a tangible effect on moving inward and "being okay" in situations where things aren't okay. Since learning it, I have heard teachers from other traditions—Buddhist, Hindu, even more open-minded Christian teachers—refer to the process in some way. Usually it's referenced simply as following the breath, but more detailed methods have helped many to change their desire to stay with a meditation practice long-term, because it just feels good and is not the punishment that they imagined.

SOME WEIRD THINGS I DO THAT REALLY HELP MY MEDITATION: A PRACTICE

There are good reasons that Patanjali didn't start the eight limbs with "Sit down, meditate and reach enlightenment." It's a process, which is the basis of *Hatha* yoga, where we seek to balance the *ha* (solar) *nadi* (a channel or flow of energy through the subtle body) and the *tha* (lunar) *nadi.* We do *asana* to open our nostrils and energy channels to help our focus so we can move inward.

As much as I adored my teacher Easwaran, he didn't give us (his students) much instruction to prepare for seated practice. He told us to sit up straight and take *mantram* walks during the day to keep our bodies strong for sitting. Though I learned much under his brilliant tutelage, rarely was meditation easeful for me; it always seemed like hard work.

Over the last 40 years or so, I've found some practices that not only make my meditation less arduous, but often really blissful. Maybe you'll find them to be helpful as well. The whole set of exercises below can take about 20 minutes and work best when done sequentially, but you can experiment and find the ones that work best for you.

Before you begin, check the flow of air in your nostrils (known as *swara* in Sanskrit) to see which one feels more open: close one side and breathe in and out and then check the other side. Note the difference. You may find this interesting, as which nostril breathes with more ease is said to reflect your brain's hemisphere dominance (right nostril connected to left hemisphere, and left nostril connected to right hemisphere), and some say it also reflects the state of the nervous system. Many meditators express having feelings of greater mental clarity and calm when the nostrils are balanced.

TIPTOE PUSHUPS

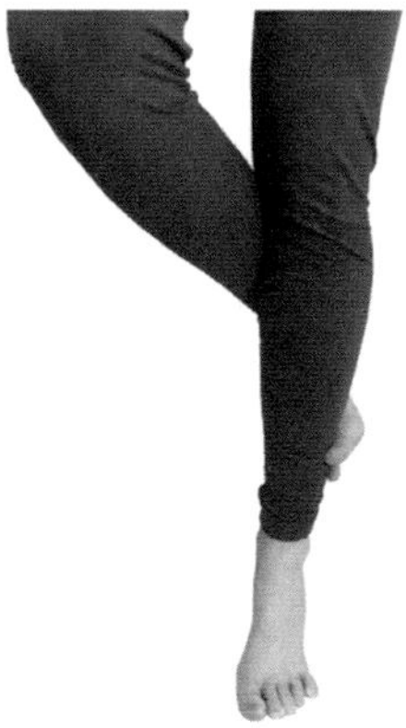

Being distracted by "sleeping" feet can be a problem in meditation, and I find that this practice helps to keep mine "awake." Plus it really strengthens the arches of the feet and helps with moving the feet into a comfortable seated posture.

Stand on one foot and do 10 heel raises. Then switch sides. You can rest a hand on a wall or chair for support.

THOPPUKARANAM (HANDS-TO-EARS *KRIYA*, ALSO KNOWN AS "SUPERBRAIN YOGA"!)

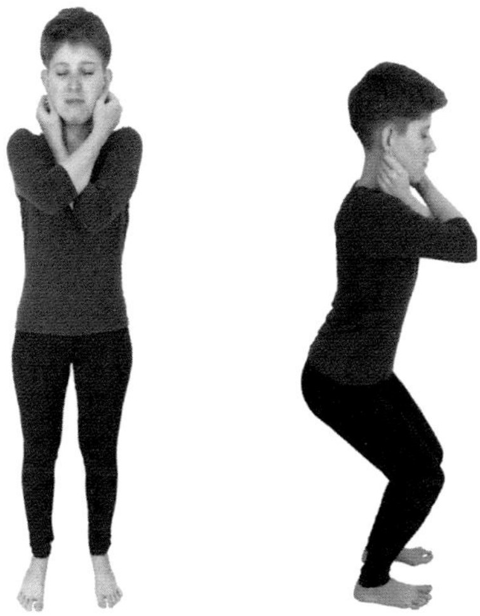

This practice helps on so many levels! It strengthens the gluteal and lower back muscles and tones the pelvic floor, which can help you to maintain alignment in your seated meditation practice; bringing the hands to the ears stimulates the pineal and pituitary acupressure points; plus, it involves crossing the midline, which research shows helps brain function.[5]

If desired, place a block on its narrowest setting between your shins for this one—this helps to keep your knees and pelvis aligned. Begin in *Tadasana* (Mountain Pose). Avoid locking your knees. Bring your left hand to your right earlobe and your right hand to your left earlobe, and squeeze gently. Inhale and squat (like you would for Chair Pose), and exhale as you rise, keeping your elbows lifted so you don't round forward. Start with 18 repetitions (you can work up to as many as 108).

Now check the balance in your nostrils again. Is the blocked side more open? It's pretty surprising how well *Thoppukaranam Kriya* works!

LATERAL STRETCH

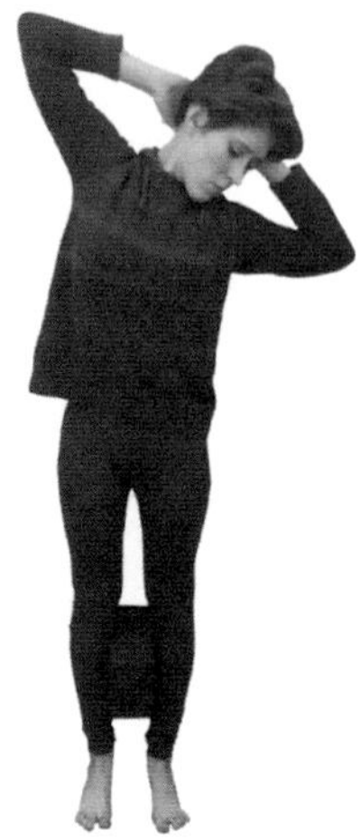

Place a block between your shins, interlace your hands behind your head, and press your head into your hands. On an exhale, side bend to the right and hold this lateral stretch for 3 breaths, breathing into your ribs; then switch sides. The ribcage holds a lot of tension, and lateral stretches can also help with vagus nerve tone (the cranial nerves that communicate to all our visceral organs that we aren't in danger), so we can relax.

TWISTED *AGNI SARA* (FIRE ESSENCE)

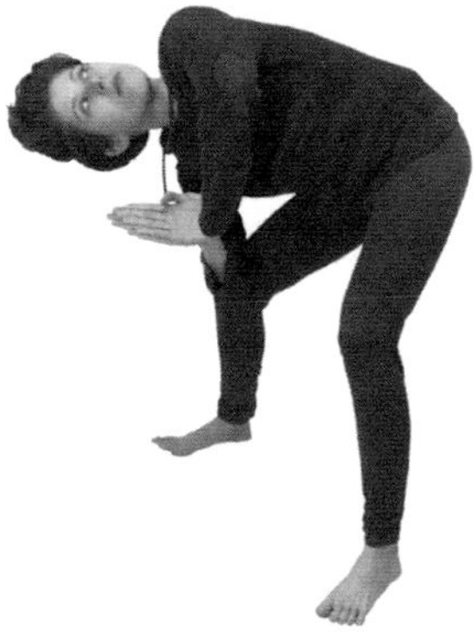

Waking up the belly brain is a good way to improve focus. We know that the microbes in the gut affect mental stability, and meditation is all about mental stability.

Stand with your feet a bit more than hip width apart, and bring your hands into *Anjali Mudra* (Prayer Position) with your elbows wide. Bend your knees until when you twist you can take your right elbow to your right knee without rounding your back, gazing down toward the floor. On an exhale, contract your pelvic floor and lower abdomen as you turn your face upward and shift your left shoulder back. Inhale as you look down, untwisting slightly. Do 3 repetitions. (If you experience lightheadedness, decrease the abdominal contraction.) Return to your starting position, take 3 breaths, then switch sides.

SCAPULAR ROLLS

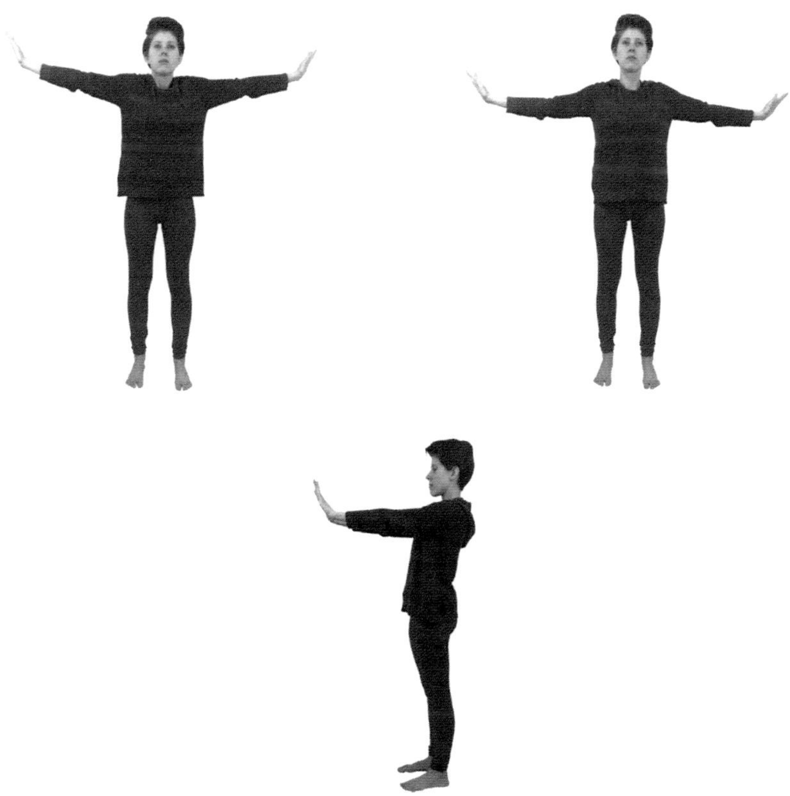

Relieving upper back tension can make for more comfortable sitting.

Stand with your arms out in a T and your wrists extended as though you were pressing your hands into walls. Move your shoulder blades every which way—forward, backward, in, out—as you breathe deeply. Then, reach your arms straight out in front of you, still extending your wrists so that your palms face forward, and roll your shoulder blades in all directions from this position.

ARM SWINGS

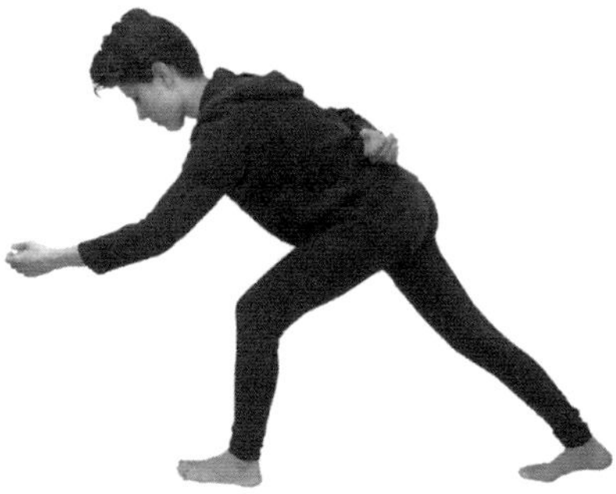

This practice has a "cooling" effect on the shoulder capsule, which can be very calming. I find that it seems to deepen my breath after the practice (which is useful for meditation). Perhaps this is because of the effect it is said to have on the heart and lung meridians that run down the inner and outer arms.

From Mountain Pose, step your left foot forward and bend your left knee, as in Warrior I, though your back heel may be off the floor. Bring your right forearm behind your waist and hinge forward from your hips, keeping your spine long. Swing your left arm like an elephant's trunk (in circles, figure 8s, or whichever way your arm swings), using momentum rather than muscular control, for 3–5 breaths. Then reach your left arm up toward the ceiling, step your feet together, lower your arms to your sides, and switch sides.

Of course, you don't need to do all of these things. It seems that the type of movement that makes a difference for someone—that will open up a nostril that is "shut down"— depends on where they have their energetic blockages. For some people, even jaw hinge release or throat opening work like Lion's Breath or the Singing Snake (Moorcha) exercise described on page 107 can help with feeling the breath in both sides. Unblocking the flow of breath through the nostrils is an important step for any of the *Prana Dharana* methods that follow.

PRANA DHARANA METHODS

Method 1

PHASE 1

Come to an upright seated posture. Do a circular *Nadi Shodhana*: Slowly inhale through your left nostril and exhale through your right nostril 3 times. Rest for 3 breaths, then inhale through your right nostril and exhale through your left nostril for 3 rounds. Rest in breath awareness after the third round.

You can do multiple cycles of this, but just one is often pretty effective if you're short on time. This helps sensitize the area of the nostrils to which you are bringing attention.

PHASE 2

Relax into abdominal breath, feeling the nuances of your breath dropping down below your ribcage.

Then, without changing the relaxed way you are breathing, bring awareness to the feeling of your breath moving through your chest. Draw your attention to the passage of air through your throat; at this point feel the coolness of your breath entering your body and the warmth of your breath leaving your body.

Now feel the subtlety of your breath in your nostrils, brushing in and out.

Then bring awareness to only the upper part of your nostrils, following a line up the interior nostrils to the point between your eyebrows. Draw that line deeper into your head as though forming an arc from the tip of your nose to the center of your head (the midbrain around the hypothalamus, the thalamus, the pituitary and pineal area (the pranic hub)). Maintain a steady flow of breath and pay attention to its subtlety.

A *mantra* such as *so-ham* or a personal *mantra* can accompany the breath if desired.

Method 2

Phase 1

Begin again with a breath practice. *Bhastrika* (Bellows Breath) is often effective in waking up the nasal sensitivity. This is done with strong exhalation and inhalation emanating from the abdomen at a pace that allows for a complete inhalation and exhalation (often around 50 rounds per minute).

If you feel dizzy or the Bellows Breath feels uncoordinated, you can use the alternate nostril practice above.

Phase 2

Drop into relaxed diaphragmatic breathing, with attention to the bottom rim of your nostrils (the area closest to your lips).

Move your attention to the outer rim of each nostril, as though the breath were flaring your nostrils on the inhalation and relaxing them on the exhalation.

Bring attention to the sensations of your breath brushing the interior rim of your nostrils and septum.

Now, feel your breath along the upper nasal membranes, gathering more and more sensitivity to both directions of the breath, both in and out, and lift that awareness as though it were sweeping the frontal lobe of your brain. After sitting with this consciousness of breathing for a few minutes, focus your mind on an inspirational or scriptural passage or *mantra* to help hold your attention.

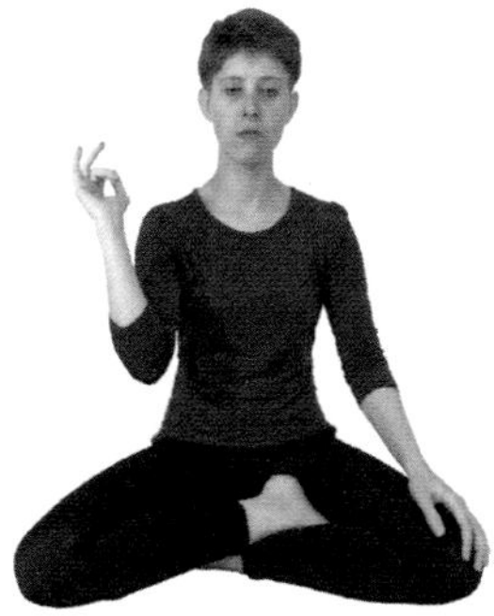

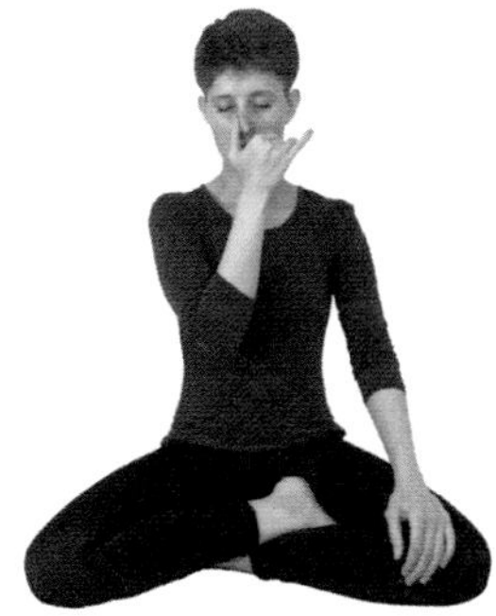

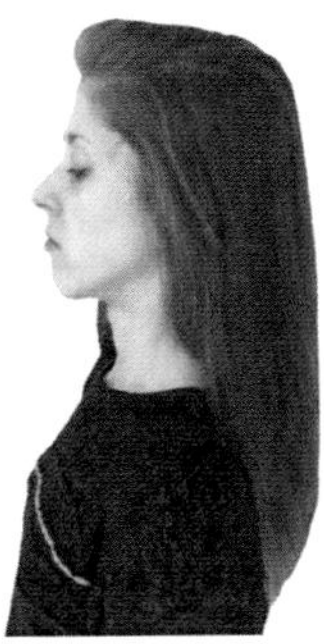

Method 3

PHASE 1

This time, for an alternate nostril practice, use the same weight of inhalation and exhalation with the abdominal contraction on exhalation as in *Bhastrika*. This practice is called *Surya Bhedi* (Sun-Piercing Breath).

With your ring finger, block the flow of breath lightly just below the nose cartilage in your left nostril; then through your right nostril exhale-inhale-exhale-inhale. Now switch sides, blocking the flow of your right nostril with your thumb and exhale-inhale-exhale-inhale through your left nostril. Do this 10 times on both sides.

After the tenth round, take a long inhalation through your right nostril. Hold it briefly and release slowly.

Repeat starting on the left side and end with a long inhalation through your left nostril after the tenth round.

Phase 2

Begin with long relaxed abdominal breathing until the rhythm of your breath is steady and the inhalation and exhalation are balanced in length and quality.

Focus on the temperature in your right nostril as your breath moves in and out of it.

Refine your awareness down to the finest line of where you feel coolness on the way in and warmth on the way out.

Locate the point where your breath changes temperature.

Now do the same in your left nostril, really refining a sense of location of temperature change and minute refinement.

Bring your awareness to both nostrils, attempting to feel very balanced between both hemispheres of the brain and with a sense of brain synergy for your meditation practice—even the attempt to feel this balance can leave one very refreshed.

CHAPTER 5

Viva la Vagus!

You know that great feeling you get from a super stretchy yawn? Or how about that anticipation right before a sneeze, when you know it's going to be a really good one? Those are vagus nerve sensations and there is tons of new information out there about this rock star of cranial nerves.

"*Vagus*" is the Latin word for "wandering," and indeed this bundle of nerve fibers roves through the body and is the connection between the brain and the major organs as well as other nerves that are involved in speech, eye contact, facial expressions, and even the ability to tune in to other people's voices. It is made of thousands of fibers, 80 percent of which are sensory, meaning that the vagus nerve's connection doesn't just listen to the brain but reports back from your organs to your brain. We are learning more and more about what an essential element the vagus is to the parasympathetic nervous system and to our health in general (it calms the adrenal response and gives the organs the "okay" to do the work they do when there is no immediate danger to the organs).

A study at Boston University School of Medicine demonstrated evidence that vagal tone might be the reason we feel better, blissed, and blessed after a yoga practice.[1] The American Medical Association (AMA) has labeled poor vagal tone as a symptom of legions of health issues, but yoga might view it as a *cause*. Doctors have discovered that a vagus nerve stimulation procedure, involving the implantation of a device that stimulates the vagus nerve with electrical impulses, helps control the symptoms of people with epilepsy and medication-resistant depression. The nerve has even been severed surgically to diminish appetite for weight loss! Fortunately, this practice is no longer in vogue.

Through practices unique to yoga—*Ujjayi* Breath, *Prachardhana* (a husky *Bhastrika*-type breath that stimulates the soft palate and the glandular and brain area above), breath control in *Viparita Karani* (Inverted-Action Pose), *Matsyasana* (Fish Pose), *Agni Sara*, and more—the vagus receives stimulation. As a result, a systematized, therapeutic approach to *asana* (rather than a typical fitness-type yoga workout) can provide ground for deep healing to begin. While *Vinyasa* Flow Yoga or Power Yoga can cause a rise in endorphins and an ensuing feeling of calm, and fit people have overall better vagal tone, it takes a skilled teacher to make such a practice a subtle exploration of energy. I've seen it done, but rarely.

I can't help but notice that the diagrams of the vagus nerve look remarkably like the anatomy of the *chakras*. And the fact that the vagus nerve produces an altruistic bliss state when activated is very interesting indeed.

Our body naturally stimulates the vagus nerve with acts like coughing, sneezing, yawning, and bearing down for a bowel movement. Natural *pranayama*! But yoga can provide a direct boost for the parasympathetic nervous system, unlike any other form of medical treatment or "exercise." When the vagus nerve is stimulated, the parasympathetic nervous system has its day—think rest and digest, the sweet buzz of well-being.

When vagal tone is poor, organs function poorly: Our heart races and the lungs strain, and the liver, kidneys, and stomach can all suffer. Since vagus nerve stimulators are being used to treat seizures, depression, and Alzheimer's, the importance of this nerve is apparent. Poor posture and compression of the nerve exacerbate poor communication between organs and the brain. When the root issue is not addressed and only its symptoms are attacked, health typically continues to diminish.

While our "healthcare" system (read "sick care") runs around with fire hoses, Yoga Therapy and *Ayurveda* address the guy holding the matches. Here, rather than piling medicines (or supplements) on a weak digestive and immune system, we address stressors. The weakened vagus nerve needs support—not necessarily a laxative, antacid, cold pill, or myriad interventions. It does no good to kick a grumpy dog.

Don't get me wrong, there are times when the firefighters are needed and I'm grateful for lifesaving medical interventions. But the first step is to stop throwing the matches at the brittle, exhausted nervous system.

The thing to remember as we build our healthy immune and digestive systems is that when something doesn't fit, we let it go. Rewarding ourselves with the deliciousness of robust health is a gift that outweighs every indulgence.

In the winter months, I might like an icy soft drink in the afternoon as a pick-me-up, but is it worth the constipation that will likely ensue from suppressing my digestive fire? Not really. That old "choosing what is beneficial over what is pleasant" thing applies, every time. *Shreya* wins, *preya*…sorry, Man…except when it comes to stimulating vagal tone. Sweet peace—a wellspring of compassion and healthy benefits—what a deal! Many of my clients in drug and alcohol recovery have said practices that increase vagal tone are just what they've been looking for all along!

We differ in our reactions to stress and this is reflected in vagal tone. Vagal tone can be determined in part by using an electrocardiogram to measure heart rate. Your inhalation increases your heart rate to speed the flow of oxygenated blood around your body. Exhalation slows the heart rate down. Heart rate variability is one of many things regulated by the vagus nerve—the greater the variability, the higher your vagal tone. Simply changing your awareness and pattern of breath is a remarkably quick way to alter heart rate variability and gain more control over your nervous system.[2] Start by inhaling for 4 seconds and exhaling for 4 seconds, gradually building to 6 seconds in and 6 seconds out without strain, to have the most impact on the nervous system and cortisol levels.

Put Out the Fire

High vagal tone reduces the likelihood of diabetes, stroke, and cardiovascular disease, primary causes of death in the USA, all of which involve inflammation. Those with low vagal tone are more likely to suffer from inflammation of all kinds. Inflammation is useful for assisting in healing after an injury,[3] but can cause blood vessel and organ damage (see Matt's story later in this chapter) when the immune system is not functioning well. Low vagal tone means immunity is less effective and inflammation can become excessive and damaging. One of the vagus nerve's jobs is to reset the immune system and switch off production of the proteins that fuel inflammation.

I've become somewhat of a fan of Wim Hoff, known as the "Iceman" because he can withstand an ice bath for nearly two hours without losing his core temperature. Why is this even a valuable skill? Because cooling the body is one method of increasing vagal tone (it is called "cold thermogenesis"). While I am not ready to go to his extremes, nor do I recommend his high-energy breath practices for public consumption, many people can tolerate a modified version. Students of *Kundalini* Yoga are big on cold showers as well as fiery breath work—likely for the same reasons—though they may only acknowledge Breath of Fire and cold exposure as an energetic boost. Chinese Buddhists often wash their faces with cold or iced water, which has a similar effect on vagal tone. My method for taking a cold shower is to start with comfortable warm water and lower the temperature at the end, then towel off briskly.

The vagus nerve is a ticket to well-being that we are just beginning to understand for treatment of trauma and hacking the nervous system to treat and heal anxiety, depression, chronic pain, temporomandibular joint problems, gastrointestinal issues, and more. This access to the peripheral nervous system is the way to regulate and soothe the mind and the body. In my personal and professional experience, I've seen nothing else be as effective in working with fear and trauma-based issues as this breath/mind/body modality.

While current technology allows doctors to implant a vagal stimulator for certain types of intractable epilepsy and treatment-resistant depression, there's a meridian of the vagus nerve that can be accessed by stimulating the external ear. This is what acupuncturists believe allows them to influence the body more precisely than an electrode in the neck.

Many of my Yoga Therapy clients respond well to two-handed "self-unrolling" of the ear (taking both hands to one ear and gently pulling around the circumference of the ear including the hard point tragus up front), with extra pressure applied to sensitive points around the edges of the ear. Some, especially those in addiction recovery, do even better with ear acupuncture than self-acupressure, though it may not be accessible to all. (Many inpatient treatment programs now offer routine ear acupuncture.)

STRESS BUSTER PRACTICE

Below are some of the *asana* techniques I have found most helpful in stimulating vagus response. They can be practiced individually or together as a sequence. For those who are susceptible to light-headedness or dizziness, try 1 round when 3 are recommended in order to test the waters.

When I used these with people in recovery, they often expressed gratitude, explaining that the vagus techniques gave them a practice that helped with cravings and acting out, and a bit of a natural buzz to help fill the void left by substance abuse.

Do be aware that overstimulation of the vagus nerve can cause fainting (I've never seen it happen with these techniques but proceeding with caution is always a good idea).

SEATED TWIST WITH ABDOMINAL CONTRACTION

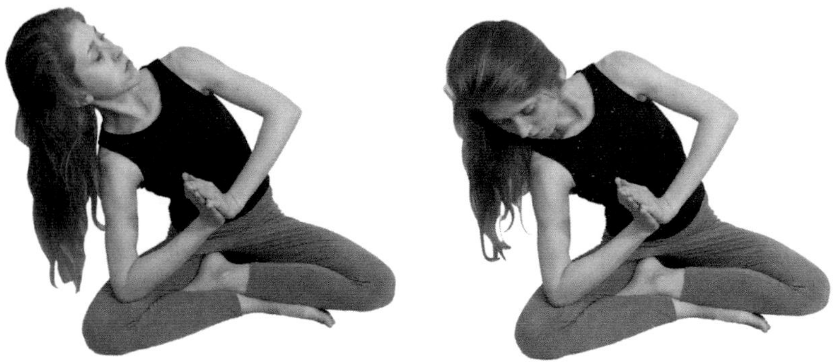

Start by learning to do the Abdominal Lift in a reclining position with your knees bent and feet on the floor: On an exhalation, lightly draw up the floor of your pelvis and your abdomen (don't be aggressive with this practice). On an inhalation release the contraction.

Once you feel comfortable with drawing up your abdomen on an exhalation, sit in a chair or in *Sukhasana* (Easy Posture). Bring your hands to *Anjali Mudra* (Prayer Position) in front of your heart and tilt to the right, taking your right elbow to your right knee, with your head in line with your spine.

Exhale and contract your abdomen and pelvic floor as you turn your chin toward your left shoulder (you can also roll your left shoulder back).

Inhale as you turn your face back to look at your right knee, releasing the contraction.

Do 3 repetitions on this side if it is comfortable and you have no dizziness. After 3 rounds, inhale back to center and sit for several breaths to feel the effect. Repeat on the other side, then relax and enjoy the relaxing buzz that follows. This technique can also be done standing in Chair Pose.

LATERAL REACH AND MELT

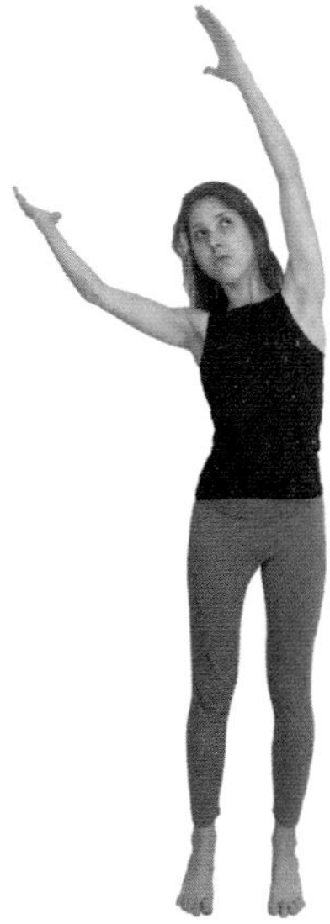 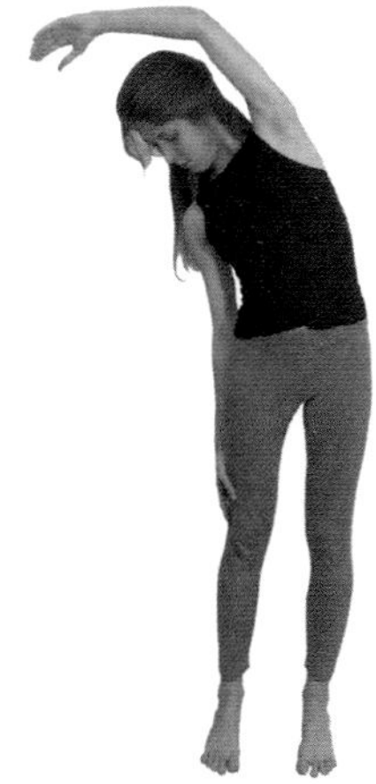

You can stand or sit in a chair or in *Sukhasana*. Take your right hand to the floor or to the edge of the chair.

Inhale, raise your left arm up and, on an exhalation, arc to the right. Then inhale and reach diagonally to the right. Exhale and bend your left elbow a little to warm up into the lateral reach.

Repeat this extension and flexion of the elbow 2 more times, then after the last reach, let your arm soften and become heavy in a soft arc over your ear. Let your face soften downward and allow your neck and face to relax. Take 3 long breaths into your left ribs.

Slowly rise back to starting position on an inhalation. Pause for 3 or more breaths before doing the practice on the other side.

DEER POSE (MERMAID) TO *BHARADVAJASANA* (TWIST DEDICATED TO THE SAGE BHARADVAJA)

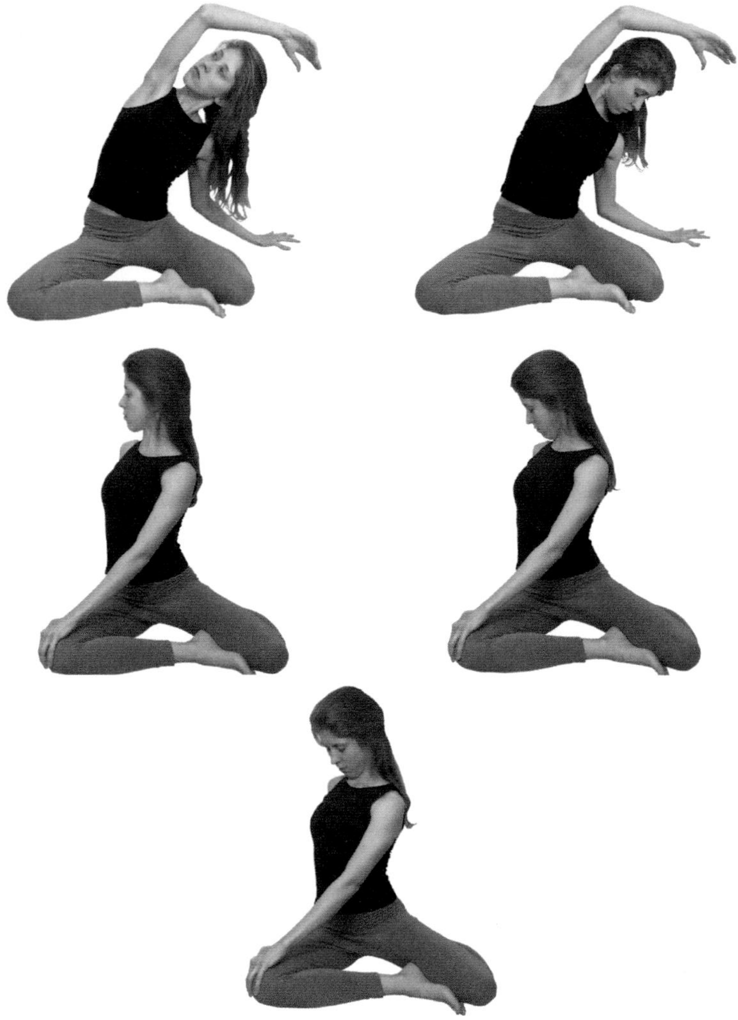

Come to a kneeling position and sit back on your heels (*Vajrasana*), then slide your hips off to the right. (You may need a folded blanket or cushion for support under your right hip in this side-saddle position.)

Inhale and raise both arms upward, then exhale as you arc to the left so your body makes a C shape. Drop your right hand to the floor, and let your body and face softly release into the curve.

After 3 breaths, slowly lift to center, then revolve your torso to the right in a twist, keeping your spine lifted.

Take your left hand to the outside of your right knee and rest your right hand behind your torso. Inhale as you lift your spine in an axial extension (spine lengthening), and use the gentle pressure of your left hand to assist in releasing your spine.

Lower your chin toward your right collarbone for 2 breaths, toward the center of your collarbones for 2 breaths and toward your left collarbone for 2 breaths.

Slowly release the pose, returning your head to center. Rest for a moment before beginning on the other side.

SINGING SNAKE AND MOORCHA (SWOONING BREATH)

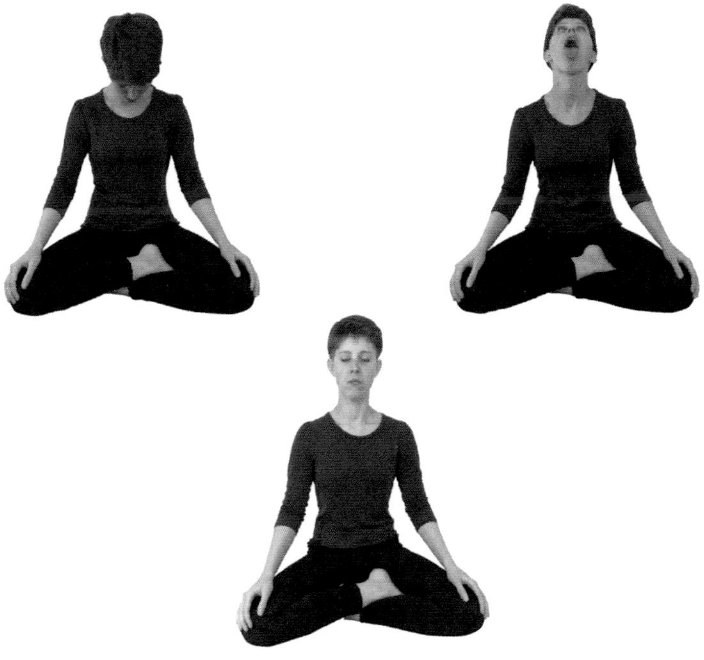

Sit in a tall, comfortable, stable position. Drop your chin toward your chest as you inhale. Exhale as you lift your chin upward, extend your tongue, and breathe out through your mouth. Then, leaving your chin up, close your mouth and inhale. Exhale slowly as you lower your chin to a neutral position. If you feel dizzy, stop. If pleasantly relaxed, you could try variations of tilting the head back slightly to the left or the right on the lift. Take it easy—3 times is likely enough.

Jaw Tension, and What to Do about It

Temporomandibular joint disorders (TMD, commonly known as TMJ for "temporomandibular joint") are some of the most common complaints of my Yoga Therapy clients (especially those with high levels of anxiety, though they often only mention TMJ after back, shoulder, and hip issues because they don't see Yoga Therapy as something that can help jaw pain or stiffness, the most troublesome of the primary symptoms of these disorders). My clients are often surprised by how much yoga has to offer when it comes to relieving tension in the jaw.

The trigeminal nerve is the fifth cranial nerve and communicates between the face and the brain. It has an ophthalmic connection (to the eye area), a maxillary connection, and a mandibular connection (these latter two affect the jaw). Sympathetic and parasympathetic fibers join the three divisions and are distributed to the pupil, to the nasal mucosa causing mucus secretion, to the lacrimal, submaxillary, and sublingual glands, and to the arterioles of the face.

Misalignment of the head, a major contributor to jaw issues, is common because of the jutting forward we do each day as we drive, look at cell phones, and work at computers. Many lines of work, such as photography or even teaching children (think leaning down to listen) promote pushing the head forward, and the more often we do this the more it becomes a body *samskara* (a deeply ingrained habit). When the head pushes forward, the jaw has to adjust, often even changing the way the teeth align, which is why this action might contribute to jaw pain or stiffness.

I was listening to a podcast recently about the societal prevalence of jaw issues and it confirmed much of what I see in my practice. The podcast also pointed to the psychological stresses as well as the impact on other cranial nerves when the trigeminal is pinched or compressed by misalignment. I have noticed the full body relief people feel when tension is lessened in the jaw hinge through the use of yoga techniques; in fact, following some dental work that shifted my bite, I am personally finding many of these techniques to be helpful and stress-relieving.

Before we explore yoga poses that can benefit the jaw, let's look first at some practical daily solutions for relieving jaw tension.

- Be mindful throughout the day to draw your skull up and back and sit up straight. Sounds simple, but it's a remembering game. Getting your computer off your lap and walking while leading with your chest instead of your nose are a couple of examples of mindful ways to make sure your head isn't jutting forward.

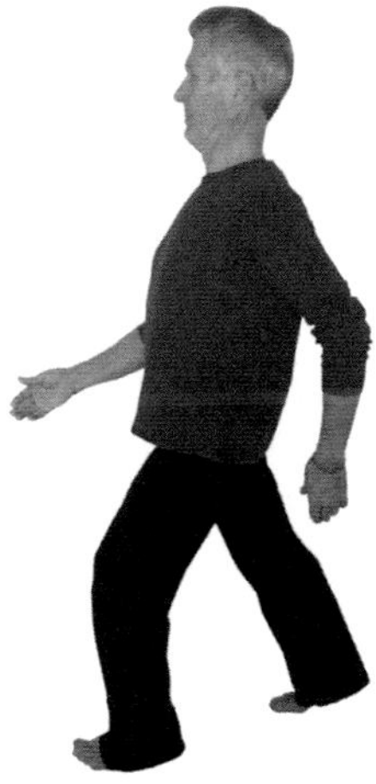

- Take jaw breaks and try to circle your jaw using your hand and not your jaw muscles a few times a day to release mandibular tension.

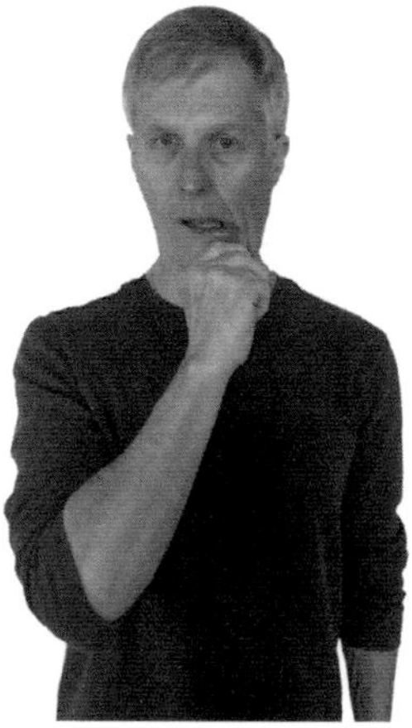

- Bring your head into an up and back position, then roll your tongue around the front of your teeth 10 times in each direction.

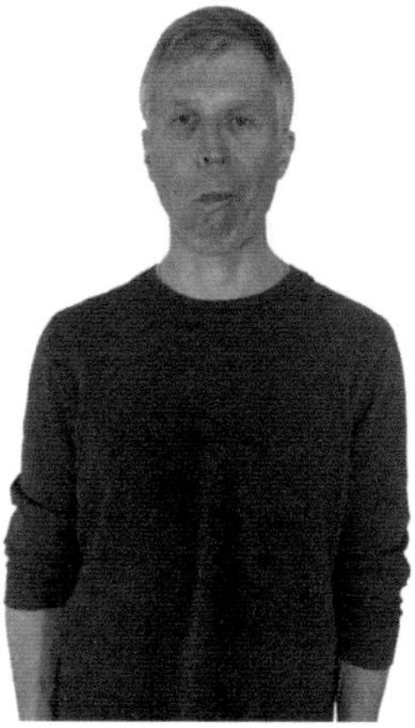

A YOGA PRACTICE FOR JAW TENSION

Here, we can rediscover how we may have been harboring jaw tension and how we can best release it. Do the short practice that follows before bed to help your jaw heal.

VAMPING POSE

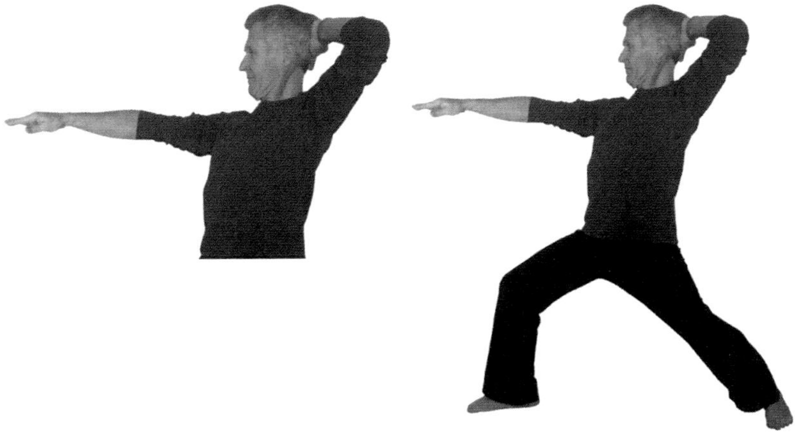

While seated, cup the base of your skull with your left hand, and slightly lengthen the back of your neck. Then reach your right arm out to the side (like a Warrior II position). Hold for 3 breaths. Then repeat on the other side.

Cupping the base of the skull like this can serve as a reminder of how royal we feel when we get the head centered, and it's something that you can do throughout your day and your yoga practice (as in Warrior II) to avoid jutting the head and jaw forward.

DOWNWARD-FACING COBRA

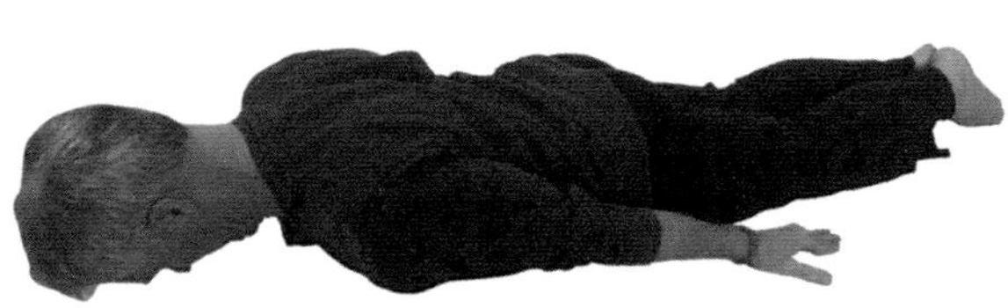

This pose can help to strengthen the back of your neck and help you with finding your optimal head alignment.

Typically, we lift our faces when practicing Cobra Pose, but for this variation, your intention is to keep your chin slightly tucked and to focus on the extension of your upper back (not your neck). Lie on your belly with your inner thighs together, your forehead hovering just above the floor, and your arms resting along your sides with palms facing down. On an inhalation, keep your gaze down and the back of your neck long as you lift your chest away from the floor. On an exhalation, release. Do 5 lifts and lowers, thinking about lifting the back of your head as you rise.

UNLOCKING THE JAW

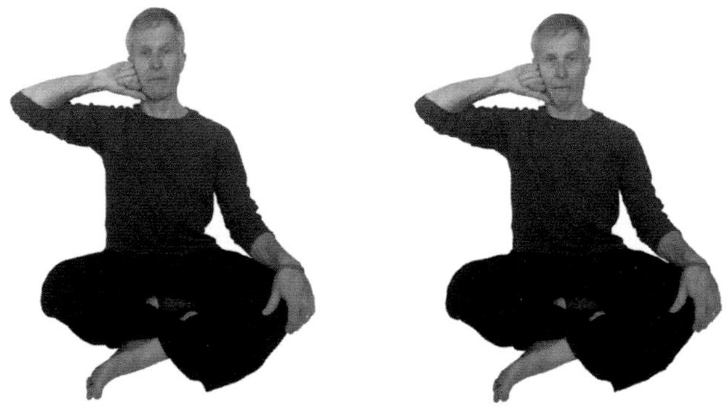

Start seated in a chair or on the floor. Place a soft fist on one side of your jaw. Without moving your hand, first try to turn your head toward your fist, engaging the sternocleidomastoid in that side of your neck.*

---

* The sternocleidomastoids in each side of the neck are responsible for rotating the head to the opposite side; working together, these muscles also flex the neck, extending the head.

Gently shift the action to the jaw itself by pressing it toward your hand, holding for 1–2 breaths and then releasing (you can open your mouth to keep the hinge more relaxed). Only press briefly, so that your jaw doesn't get inflamed or feel "poppy." Then repeat the action on the other side.

NECK STRENGTHENER

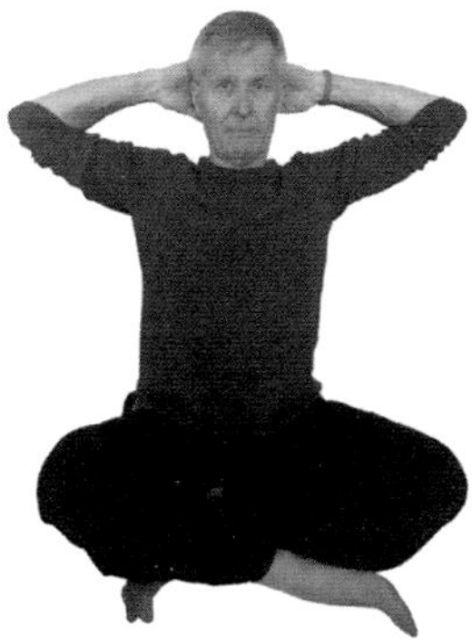

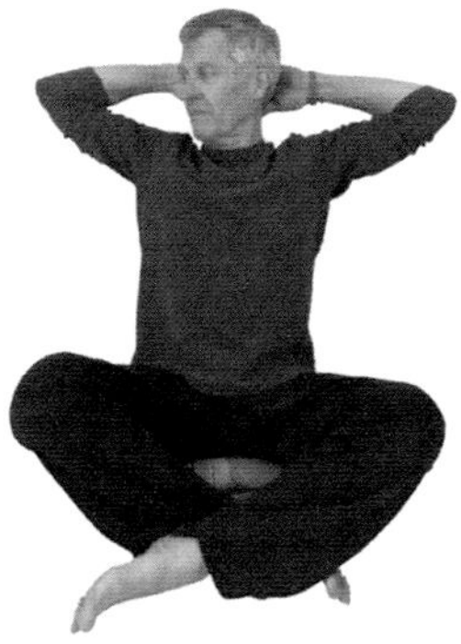

Interlace your fingers behind your head and gently press your head into your palms. Hold for 3 breaths. Then turn your head to the right and press it back into your palms for 3 breaths. Repeat on the other side.

HEAD HAMMOCK FLEXION AND CERVICAL EXTENSION

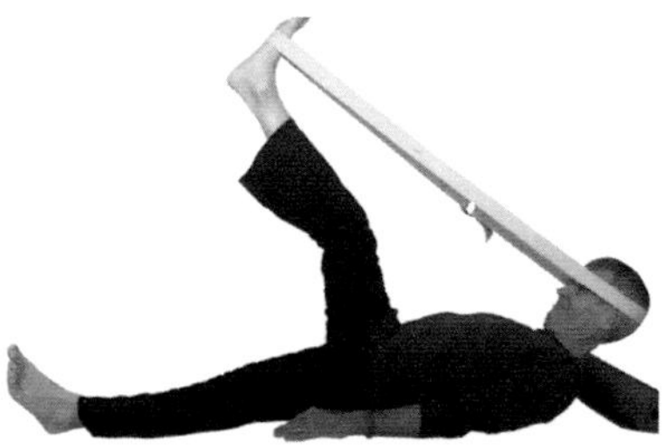
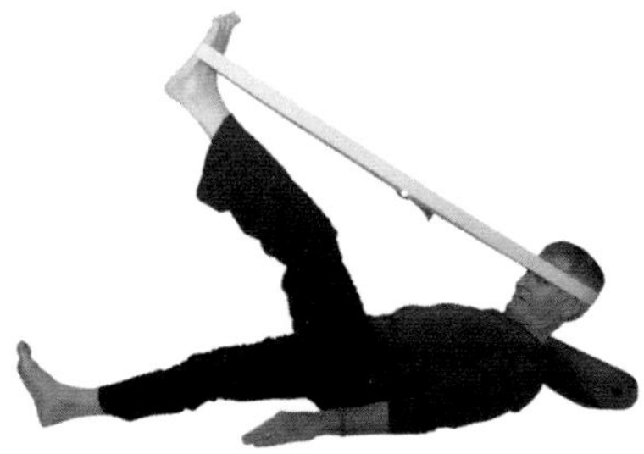
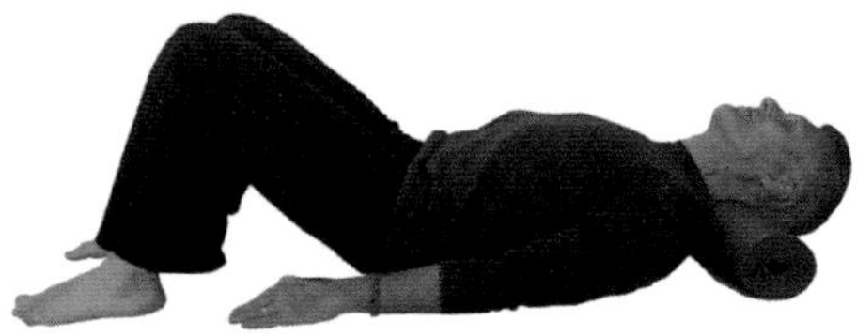
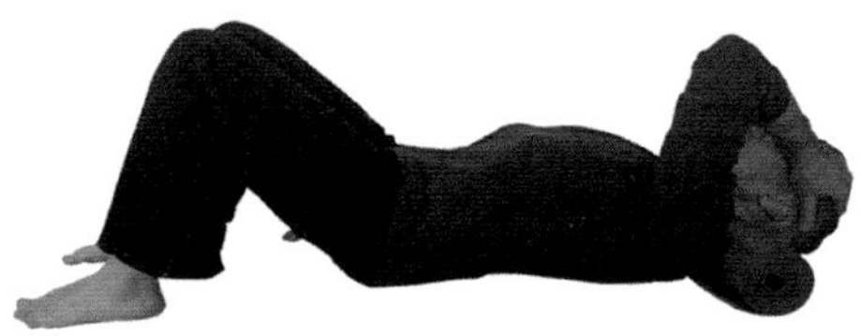
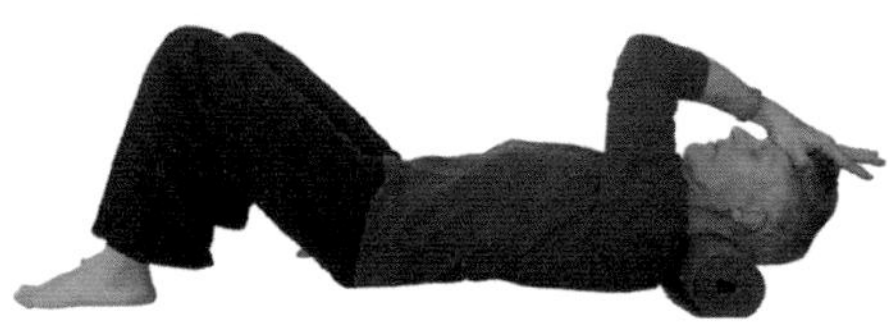

These poses will stretch first the back and then the front of the neck, areas which can feel tight for people with jaw tension.

Before you practice Head Hammock, you'll want to have your props already set up for the Cervical Extension so that you can release right back into it. To set up, make a big loop with your yoga strap (you'll want a strap that's at least 8 feet long or 10 feet long if you're over 6 feet tall); make sure that the loop is secure and keep the looped strap within arm's reach. Place an angled bolster under your thighs if you like (you can angle the bolster on blocks, though for shorter legs you may want to skip angling the bolster, especially if your feet hover above the floor) and a rolled-up sticky mat on the floor behind you, horizontally. To position yourself, lie back over the rolled mat so that it supports your neck, adjusting the placement of the roll as necessary to align the C-7 vertebra at the base of the neck with the bottom of the roll. Your head will likely not touch the floor.

Once you have your set-up, pick up the securely looped strap and wrap one end of the loop behind your head, supporting it just above your ears, and place the other end around the arch of one foot. Extend that leg toward the sky, flexing your foot, and let your head be supported by the strap. Your bottom leg can be extended or bent. Stay in this position for 2–5 minutes, then repeat on the other side. When you switch feet, you can also angle your head slightly in order to release one side of your neck and then the other.

Remove the strap and lie back over the rolled mat. Remember, you want the mat roll supporting your neck, with C-7 at the bottom of the roll and your head tilting back. Allow your jaw to relax completely. Your mouth may be open here, which can help your jaw to relax.

Gently press one hand to your forehead for 1–2 breaths to encourage your head to fully relax. Then, place your arms back down at your sides and a relaxed distance from your body and remain like this for 5 minutes.

Now bring your right hand to your right temple and briefly press into that hand. Repeat on the other side, and then bring the heel of your hand between your eyebrows and press your head to the palm lightly before removing the roll and letting your body rest in *Savasana* for several minutes before getting up.

In addition to this short yoga sequence and the tips to apply throughout the day, there's one more thing you can do for jaw tension: When you go to bed, encourage ease and relaxation in your jaw by counting out long deep breaths (4 counts or more on both your inhalation and exhalation) until you fall asleep. Relieving jaw tension may prove to be a ticket to better sleep and may lessen your stress overall so that you find that relaxing the jaw through yoga practice has a domino effect on the stress in your whole body!

Matt's Story

When Matt came in for a Yoga Therapy session, I was struck by his handsome face, charming demeanor, and his gaunt, jaundiced appearance. His palms were as yellow as bananas. He had just had a heart pacemaker installed and was on a waiting list for a liver transplant. He was a 24-year-old newlywed with a stepson he adored. Initially Matt had tried to attend a very vigorous public yoga class and tended to push a little too hard for someone going through such a crisis.

Matt and I talked about life and what had led up to this condition, which had the doctors mystified. Why organ failure at such a young age? As we chatted, Matt leaned forward to speak and listen. His compassionate mannerism of pushing his head forward had become habitual to the point that his cervical spine alignment was nearly horizontal, rather than upright and slightly curved in as is optimal for cervical alignment. Matt is quite tall and in his work as a minister he would tend to "come down to people's level" with his head to be a better listener. I've noticed this tendency in many people who work in professions of compassion.

We had several sessions working mainly on deepening the breath and developing core support. During one session Matt mentioned that his surgeon—who wanted to remove Matt's gall bladder in hopes that it might be a player in his declining organ health—had told him that he had very poor vagal tone. My question was, "What if that poor vagal tone is the cause rather than a symptom of your issues?" We started working on vagus techniques and especially on postural alignment. We can't be sure, but Matt and I assume that the compression of his posterior cervical spine was so severe, it was affecting his cranial nerves. His doctors were in disbelief at the strides he made after adding these practices.

In the process, Matt fell in love with all things yoga and went through yoga teacher training at our school. His improvement was startling and his athletic skills on the mat were just fun (and at times a little scary) to watch. A year after he began Yoga Therapy sessions, his heart health improved to such an extent that he went from using his pacemaker 99 percent of the time to 61 percent to 16 percent, and finally he was not using the device at all. His liver function returned to normal and, in spite of his life being quite stressful during that time period, Matt moved to Atlanta to graduate divinity school and to become a popular yoga teacher at a large studio.

Maintaining his health requires vigilance (and he has to pay careful attention to his diet), but he has his life back and continues to heal. His interest in, and experience with, the healing power of the vagus nerve plays a powerful role in his teaching.

Helping Clients Stay Present

Writing about trauma, Bessel van der Kolk, MD, said:

> Now, many people who don't know a lot about trauma think that trauma has something to do with something that happened to you a long time ago. In fact, the past is the past and the only thing that matters is what happens right now. And what is trauma is the residue that a past event leaves in your own sensory experiences in your body and it's not that event out there that becomes intolerable but the physical sensations with which you live that become intolerable and you will do anything to make them go away."[4]

Helping a client who has experienced trauma to reassociate with their body via yoga practices can be pivotal. Recent studies show that just simply teaching them mindfulness-based practices is often unsuccessful. In a 2014 podcast, van der Kolk asserts that people who have experienced trauma have lousy heart rate variability, which is the indicator of poor vagal tone. They lose the sense of goodness and safety in the body. Trauma lands in the amygdala, which he compares to a smoke detector of the brain. Trauma makes that part of the brain hypersensitive or renders it insensitive and numb.[5] When people who have experienced trauma simply try to become silent and move inward, they often become overwhelmed and flee. That's because in mindfulness practices, we are confronted with the internal world, and the client may lack the tools to cope with the sensations that occur when that happens, and dissociation can occur.

Dissociation could also happen with Restorative or *Yin* Yoga or even massage. That's why when working with people who have experienced trauma, I like to start with more playful game-like work and move gradually toward the quieter, more meditative practices. When working one on one, it's easier to watch the eyes and breath to determine if the student is becoming stressed by "too much quiet."

Because a client may have spent years fleeing from sensations and using anything they can find to suppress those sensations, the use of cross-patterning (crossing the midline with one or more parts of the body or asking one side of the body to do something that doesn't mirror the other side) and vagal stimulation techniques (like the ones found on pages 104–108) can be quite helpful in restoring healthy function to organs and tissues. Also, the release of muscular tension that can result from basic *asana* is a boon to reconnection with the body. Eventually, the ability to move inward becomes more accessible.

CHAPTER 6

Issues in the Tissues

Fascia is a body-wide tensional network that consists of fibrous collagenous soft connective tissue. Its architecture is shaped by tensional strain, not compression. Yoga Therapy clients often find relief from mobilizing the fascia, and begin to gain an understanding of how yoga can help with discomfort and stress-related tightness in these tissues. But on a more holistic level, we suspect that fascia is the physical manifestation of memory and fears that are seemingly stored in the soft tissues of the body, and fascia is much more than the glue or fibers that hold us together. We don't yet know how, but ask your bodyworker or yoga teacher how many times emotions and memory erupt from deep tissue work in areas of a client's body. It happens all too frequently to ignore.

My clients often report that fear is tangible in injured areas of their bodies, and recently I have experienced this in my body as well. After a nasty fall on the ice last winter, which resulted in a reconstruction of my humerus and months of therapy, I would look out at the Pennsylvania snow and ice and feel the tissues of the injured arm contract and ache as though reliving the trauma. Many of my clients have recounted seeing a vehicle or a person that reminded them of a past physical trauma and experiencing pain at their site of past injury.

Along with words like "muscle memory" and "cellular memory," which have become a part of many yoga teachers' vocabulary, meet "myofascial memory." These are the tissues holding patterns, the tug that makes one side of your pelvis a little higher or keeps a shoulder from its full range of motion. After all, fascia glues us into our recognizable form of appearance every day. Its very job is to remember, for better or for worse.

Thanks to magnetic resonance imaging (MRI) and computerized tomography (CT) scans, we have come to understand that the fascia's work is much more than holding muscles, organs, and bones in place. It is actually electrically conductive. Fascia communicates. This is further understood by the accidental discovery of an organ called the interstitium, which is described as a dense layer of connective tissues found throughout and surrounding nearly the whole body, or a "widespread, macroscopic, fluid-filled space within and between tissues." According to Neil Theise, MD, professor in the Department of Pathology at NYU Langone Health, the protein bundles seen in this space are likely to generate electrical current as they bend with the movements of organs and muscles, and may play a role in techniques like acupuncture.

It's obviously no coincidence that the age-old teachings of yoga have spoken of such paths of energy. Now science recognizes what was once held in skepticism as a massive organ and its communication system.

Traditional Chinese Medicine refers to fascia's energetic lines of communication as meridians, while yoga and *Ayurveda* call them *nadis*, but they are essentially the same. Blockage in these energetic lines in the body can set up disturbances that can manifest physically, psychologically, and emotionally. The techniques of acupuncture, *Tai Chi*, yoga *asana* (especially *Yin* forms), massage, EFT and *Qigong* are just some of the ways humans endeavor to wake up or unlock the flow of energy. One of my favorite practices that produces tangible benefits in a short time is *Spandana*.

SPANDANA AND TECHNIQUES TO ENCOURAGE SPANDA (THE SACRED SHIVER)

The methodology of *Spandana* comes from the tradition of Kashmir Shaivism, and it is meant to awaken *spanda* (the pulse that enlivens all things). *Spanda* is that quiver before a seed sprouts or an egg hatches, and we too can feel shivers of delight or an internal flutter when *prana* (the life force) comes to our aid. The practice of *Spandana* is intended, through subtle movement, to help release energetic blocks. This includes the inflammatory blockage we know as anger (*pitta*'s fear response)—which, if unaddressed, can smolder away, leaving us (and often our loved ones) scorched.

While there are a number of different techniques you can use for the practice, here are four that can help nicely to diffuse your rage.

JIGGLING ON THE BACK

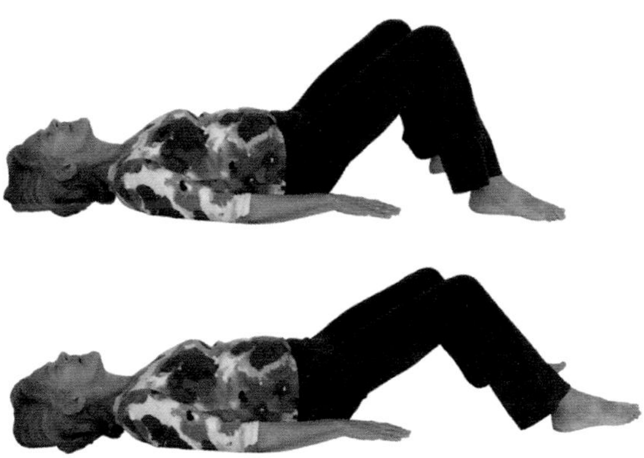

Begin in Constructive Rest Position, lying on your back with your knees bent and feet flat on the floor (experiment with the distance of your feet from your hips to find what works best for you). Slide up and down on the skin of your back, head to tailbone, with a small jiggling motion that is initiated by gently pushing intermittently with the feet (the amount of movement will differ from person to person). After about 1 minute of jiggling, rest and enjoy the after-effects.

RABBIT KICKS

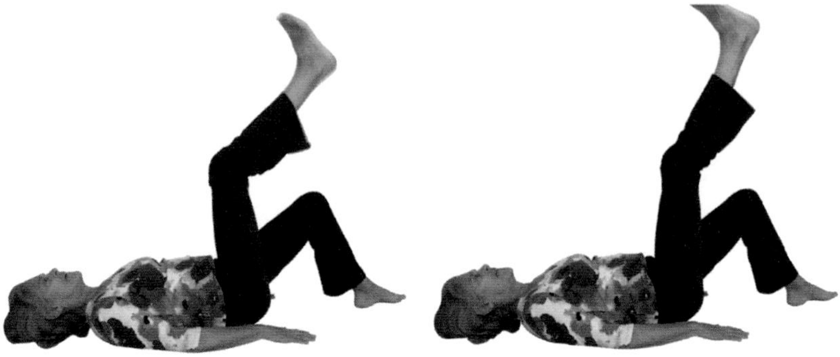

While still supine (lying on your back) in Constructive Rest Position, bring one leg up, with your knee slightly bent and your foot pointing toward the ceiling, and kick it rapidly (you can heel-kick or let the foot flop). Jiggle your leg this way for about 1 minute, and then release it back to Constructive Rest. As you release tension from that angry hip, notice the difference between the two sides. Then repeat with the other leg.

SHAKE A BIG JAR OF LEMONADE

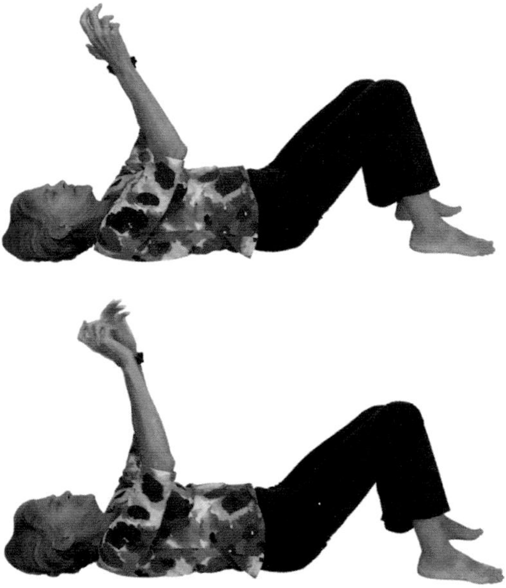

Still resting on your back, extend your arms straight up from your chest, palms parallel, as though you were holding a big jar of lemonade. Then shake as though still holding the jar, creating little shivers in your arms to release all that shoulder tension. Continue this way for 1 minute. (I like to vocalize with an "Ahhhhh" while I do this, and I usually end up laughing!)

TANTRUM

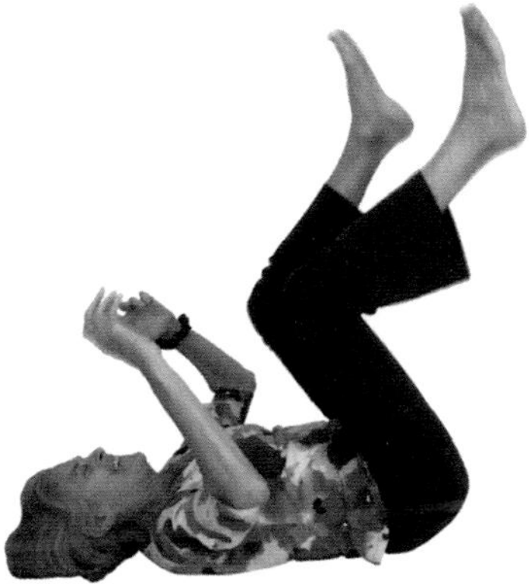

Shake everything and yell if it feels right.

Now check in with yourself and see if you're a little more able to cope with whatever came your way prior to the practice. The issue or problem that angered you may still be real and present, but how you show up to deal with it makes a lot of difference. These little practices are powerful in their ability to dissipate the anger as well as anxiety.

CHAPTER 7

Post-Traumatic Stress Disorder and How Pat-a-Cake Can Make You Brave

Rethinking Trauma and How We Address Trauma in New Ways

Dr. Hans Selye, an endocrinologist credited with pioneering studies on the effects of stress on the human body, introduced the idea of the fight/flight response back in the 1950s, and for years talk therapy was the primary method of dealing with trauma.[1] In talk therapy the idea is to get to the root of the trauma and it wasn't uncommon to re-traumatize the client by summoning the triggers for flashbacks.

While postulated by psychiatrist Pierre Janet in the late 1800s and later by Freud, it wasn't until recent years that the idea of freezing or "feigned death," as we see in possums and lizards, was accepted in the field of human psychology.[2] The recognition put forth by van der Kolk,[3] American psychologist and author Peter Levine,[4] and many of the newer breed of neuro-informed psychologists, states that trauma can stop us in our tracks and is held in the body and more primitive brain. A neuropsychotherapist, or neuro-informed psychologist, is a psychotherapist who is grounded in a sound knowledge of the neurobiological underpinnings of mental states and behavior, and whose psychotherapeutic interventions are based on or enhanced by neurobiological, cognitive, emotional, social, and environmental information.

Some of the early Rolfers and Feldenkrais and Bioenergetic therapists began to see that working with the body was an important key to helping people with post-traumatic stress disorder (PTSD). Then, as neuroscience continued to evolve, other non-verbal therapies, such as Eye Movement Desensitization and Reprocessing (EMDR), EFT (tapping), and hypnosis, were introduced as complementary therapeutic treatments for PTSD—and with some success![5]

Current thinking is that PTSD is not so much a right or left brain issue but is related to the prefrontal cortex, the limbic brain, and the lower, more primitive brain and brainstem (the culprit in that "freeze" response), and that primal response overrides the higher frontal brain.

Enter yoga, and its effect on vagal response. The shutdown (inability to feel) is vagus on overload. Remember, yoga can help with regulation of that vagal response. Yoga therapy offers a sensory-motor approach in conjunction with trauma therapy. Those in the field now understand that integrative movement can help to relieve the cycles of shame and hopelessness that accompany trauma.

According to psychologist Peter Levine, a leading proponent of somatic therapies, an interesting facet of those who endured the tragedies of 9/11 but were trapped or unable to move or help someone, was that they were more likely to experience PTSD than those who could run, react, escape, or help others effectively. Those who could not physically act were more prone to the flashbacks, the sleep difficulty, the poor memory, the feeling of a shortened future, the hypervigilance, the extreme startle response. The physical movement during the traumatic event helped the brain process and react in more functional ways.[6] According to Levine: "Trauma is not caused by the event itself, but rather develops through the failure of the body, psyche, and nervous system to process adverse events."[7]

To liken the psychological condition of PTSD to a physical state, if you have ever experienced frozen shoulder (adhesive capsulitis) you will know the pain of trying to move your shoulder past a certain range without experiencing a lot of pain. What has happened is that dense fascia has built up around the capsule of the shoulder, and the pain is prohibitive enough that it is tempting to give up and let go of the full range of motion. Movement can become more and more limited. Often the condition is a result of physical trauma, such as an accident or a fall.

From a yogic perspective, the same thing happens in emotional trauma. The memory of our abuse or grief is painful and to move into it more deeply sends a message to stop. This "frozen" memory is locked in the non-verbal right hemisphere of the brain, which is masterful at processing space and feeling, but not time—that is the left hemisphere's job. Therefore, the sensations of the memories stay in the present (flashbacks being a classic example). The underlying trauma and its symptoms are in the primitive brain, while the memory of that event is less accessible to the linear left brain.

Often, talk therapy and attempts at meditation can throw the individual into more sensation related to traumatic pain, because the pain continues to be like that frozen shoulder: "If I push into it, it hurts more. Can't I just leave it alone?" The method I have found most effective in helping people get to a place where they can feel safer moving into a greater "range of motion," and perhaps eventually be able to benefit more from therapy and meditation because they don't feel as triggered, is cross-patterning (movements that cross the midline in the body or encourage differing movement on either side). Why? Because it is sensory-motor/neural work, allowing both hemispheres of the brain to put the trauma in the plane of time (a linear function of the left hemisphere). It also has the capacity to connect the student to more primitive and even childlike movement. There are similarities to EMDR, which uses eye movements to help reduce stress around memories of the event(s). Physical cross-patterning is totally client-controlled and uses the whole body and nervous system to regain full "range of motion" (as it were).

Should All Yoga Be Trauma Sensitive?

Below is an overview of Trauma-Sensitive Yoga information that first appeared on *Yoga International*. I'll detail some cross-patterning techniques at the end of this chapter.

- Each year, about 8 million adults around the world experience PTSD. Approximately 7–8 percent of the global population will develop PTSD at some point in their lives—about 10 percent of women, and 4 percent of men.
- One in eight soldiers returning from active combat suffers from PTSD, while less than half of them seek help.
- One in five women and one in 71 men have been raped at some point in their lives. One in four girls and one in six boys will be sexually traumatized before the age of 18. (Sexual trauma is defined as any lingering physical, emotional, or psychological symptoms resulting from physical assault of a sexual nature or battery of a sexual nature.)
- In addition, 2.9 million cases of child abuse are reported each year in the USA alone.

After researching and writing about this information, I had to look hard again at the statistics. The word "sobering" simply does not describe adequately their effect on me. So much trauma.

PTSD varies in spectrum and quality, with a wide array of symptoms, which range from emotional distance and social avoidance, to violent or self-destructive outbursts, loss of memory, and flashbacks.

The classes of yoga teachers are not generally populated with tranquil, meditative cave dwellers or those who have danced through life unscathed. We don't know the backstories of our students, and they may never tell us. It is our job to develop an appropriate degree of awareness and sensitivity to emotional triggers in the yoga classroom.

The Teacher's Role

First, it is not within the scope of practice of a classroom yoga instructor to rout out the source of a student's trauma on the mat or in guided meditations. Unless one has the credentials and training to counsel, there is the potential of doing more harm than good. The same is true when offering advice with respect to treatment, and especially medications.

Second, permission to touch is to be granted by each individual. A well-intended adjustment can be a strong trigger for those in recovery from abuse. If you are touching students in a classroom, ask at the beginning of class for an okay in the form of a head nod. Consent cards or a coin at the top of each mat is another method, with tails indicating a student's preference for no adjustment. We also must not assume that because someone was fine with touch in prior classes, they're fine with it now.

My tenets on touch in yoga class have changed over the years. I have known students who were physically or emotionally injured by a casual physical adjustment from "master teachers." The truth is that no teacher can know why your knee is slightly bent, or how far your body will move in a side bend. And when you add a history of physical trauma into the mix, there is a definite need for communication between student and teacher that a public class does not afford. Slow-paced verbal skills can go far in maintaining safety. (Rescuing a student from potential injury with gesture or touch if they aren't responding to verbal cues may be an exception.)

When I began working in addiction recovery, where the incidence of associated abuse and trauma were much higher, there was little training in Trauma-Sensitive Yoga available. I saw firsthand what could cause non-participation, tears, or anger, and often when I least expected it. In these classes I learned to begin with breath-centered movement, rather than stillness (since being asked to be quiet and lie still could have links to past traumatic events). Poses such as Downward-Facing Dog, Tabletop, and Happy Baby were often met with intentionally crass wisecracks in the group:

"That's what my old man liked," or "This is how I got pregnant—again." The class would laugh nervously, and I'd have to remind myself that I wasn't in studio etiquette land anymore.

Asanas such as Child's Pose and Crocodile—where students were face down with eyes closed, and often with legs spread—were not well tolerated, especially by those having experienced sexual trauma.

To avoid all of these basic postures may not be possible. But I found that sequencing them later in the practice, when some degree of trust has been established, helps students tolerate them better.

There may be a reason for an individual choosing to practice toward the back of the classroom. If a student is concerned about having others see them from behind, I try to respect that. Those who might not agree to a Downward Dog or a Forward Fold at the front of a class are often fine near a wall.

Straps can be a trigger for both rape and abuse victims who have been bound or beaten, as well as IV drug users who may associate them with tourniquets. While they are common in most yoga studios and gyms, it may be a good idea to keep them out of view unless in use. When straps are used, I've found it to be less threatening to demonstrate clearly what we're going to do with them, and then give students the option of whether or not to use them.

Consider suggesting that students have the option of closing their eyes, rather than speaking of it as a requirement (especially for final relaxation). Hypervigilance—maintaining abnormal awareness of environmental stimuli—is typical for a person suffering from PTSD. Such an individual may have heightened startle responses or flashbacks, and being forced to keep their eyes closed can trigger these anxiety responses. The cues "Calm the eyes," or "Leave the eyes softly open, if needed," can give students the comfort of choice.

For teachers who have taught yoga for some time, words like "anus," "genitals," and "buttocks" may sound no more loaded than "elbow joint" or "thoracic spine." But I found out the hard way that students can be emotionally re-injured by our over-familiarity with these terms when giving descriptions of practices such as *Mula Bandha* (Root Lock).

A teacher-training student of mine nearly quit training when he was asked to do a report on a senior teacher's video involving an introspective practice that described using all of the musculature of the pelvis. "My childhood sexual abuse came back. I felt probed and assaulted," he explained. We can't always avoid discussions in the classroom about *bandhas* or practices such as *Agni Sara* (which involve contraction of the floor of the pelvis and abdomen), but we can be mindful of our words. Terms like "pelvic floor," "root engagement," or "drawing upward from our root" can be less inflammatory and still convey meaning. Just being aware that everyone isn't on the same page as far as comfort with anatomical terms is concerned helps us proceed with more sensitivity.

The Benefits of Cross-Patterning

There is a lot of research on the benefits of cross-patterning and its therapeutic benefits for trauma.[8] Cross-patterning is when the limbs cross the midline of the body, often making connection to the opposite side of the torso (think Eagle Pose or Sage Twist, as well as many *Kundalini kriyas* involving swinging or crossover movements). Cross-patterning can also involve "brain gym" games, such as rolling one arm or shoulder forward while the other rolls back. Incorporating more of this type of movement in class helps all yoga students with their neurological processing and coordination—but when processing trauma, the results can be quite remarkable.[9]

Being Prepared to Help Trauma Survivors

Margaret Howard, a St. Louis-based trauma therapist and advocate for survivors of human trafficking, recommends additional training for yoga teachers:

> The more I study psychological trauma, the more I become convinced. Basic training in the biology, anatomy, and physiology of trauma phenomena should be a mandatory part of yoga teacher training and certification. Without an

> understanding of how the body itself is altered by trauma, yoga teachers may be unintentionally doing harm.[10]

But not all teachers have the resources—either because of time or finances—to do another complete training. Therapist and yoga practitioner Jamie Marich, PhD, speaks about the need for trauma sensitivity in classroom yoga:

> A yoga teacher once challenged me for being too worried about the "trauma issue," too sensitive to matters of trauma because of my perspective as a counselor. She offered, "Not everyone has been traumatized." Point taken. Not everyone has HIV or blood-borne illness either, yet in healthcare settings we take universal precautions to prevent transmission because there is enough of a risk. The same reasoning applies here—trauma is enough of an issue in the general population and simple precautions can be taken to assure optimal safety for most.[11]

Other recommendations from trauma therapists include speaking in each class about safety protocols, limiting breathing practices to shorter periods, being available to students after a class, keeping imagery clear and in the present, and avoiding assumptions about how a pose feels and affects students. More important than anything else, however, are choices—choices about touch, positioning in the class, range of motion, oils and fragrances, after-class hugs, exiting the classroom when needed, or taking water and bathroom breaks. Choices matter.

And while we cannot offer the perfect class for every student, it is part of our growth as teachers and sensitive human beings to become more aware of how our words and our actions affect those in our care. Simply remembering the trauma statistics can help keep us mindful. We are not there to pity or heal students, nor to assume authority over their individual practice. We are there as human beings who have also known suffering, to keep open the space that will help our students find their soul's way. Nelson Mandela would say that human compassion binds us the one to the other, and binds us not in a way that pities or patronizes, but in a way that changes our common human suffering into hope for the future.

As a Yoga Therapist, the responsibility runs deeper. Psychologist Bessel van der Kolk[12] says that to simply ask about a trauma story is naive because trauma is overwhelming. There are those who think that simply to be friendly is going to be the best means to helping a Yoga Therapy client, when in fact, a person who has experienced abuse may associate gestures of friendliness with betrayal. The person who is smiling and giving becomes the sexual or emotional abuser. Therefore, as a therapist a face-to-face positioning may not be best, so there is a bit of distancing from the client. Nor should the therapist, or even the yoga teacher, position themselves in front of an exit in case the student/client feels trapped.

In the last few years, therapists have received so much more scientific information about hormonal response and the nervous system. Even 15 years ago we would have doubted this information, because intuitively it seems wrong. It turns out that we don't actually need the "story" of the trauma our client experienced in order to help them process. We can watch a Yoga Therapy client's movement, their eyes, and their integration of movement to find a way through their personal trauma experience (not to mention that talk therapy is not the primary role of the Yoga Therapist).

Van der Kolk emphasizes that trauma sits in one's automatic reactions and dispositions, and influences how one interprets the world, and that the goal is to help the survival brain reinterpret how one thinks. Is this yoga's realm? Well, certainly not for individuals who are solely interested in Instagram selfies and the perfection of phenomenal poses; but in the areas of cross-patterning, breath practice, and therapist/student relationship, I would say, "Yes, it is."

Thich Nhat Hanh worked with many people fleeing combat on refugee boats where there was great uncertainty. On those boats there were occasionally people who were monks or those with very deep interior practice. Thich Nhat Hanh reported that people around such individuals seemed calm. Conversely, when there was a chaotic or angry individual on the boat, those who were around such a person became more agitated and the trauma of the situation was heightened.

A Yoga Therapist must have the capacity to center and be calm in order to do effective work. Therefore, applying the principles of Yoga Therapy to oneself is essential to our work.

Both with depression and trauma there is often the thought that one will keep living the same old terrible situation. This is where yoga and movement can help open the nervous system to new options and help us escape from the same circumstances—to move beyond that collapse of the future where one keeps living the trauma again and again.

It may be a good idea to ask a client, "When will we know you are done with Yoga Therapy?" Bill O'Hanlon, LMFT, recommends that we help the client move outside of current sensations and see what comes next so they begin to see outside of the current fearful, anxious, or sad state.[13]

Sometimes just asking a client to stand in an empowered way, for example like Wonder Woman or Superman, can help them access the present. They are not their disempowered or abusive past; they have a solid ground upon which to stand. Warrior, Goddess, and strong standing balances can offer stability in practice especially when a client is being asked to embody the boldness and sturdiness of these stances. It is also beneficial for them to be allowed to go inward, head bowed in *Namaskara* (Prayer Pose), following such broad and empowering poses, as a way of physically taking in their effects.

Cross-Patterning Exercises

The spirit in which we move has a direct effect on how our body receives practice. The spirit of cross-patterning is one of levity. Below is a set of cross-patterning movements that not only help neural processing, but are a fun challenge. I enjoy seeing clients laugh during practice. If they enjoy themselves, they are more likely to practice at home.

SUPINE PRACTICE

KNEE SWIVELS WITH BLOCK

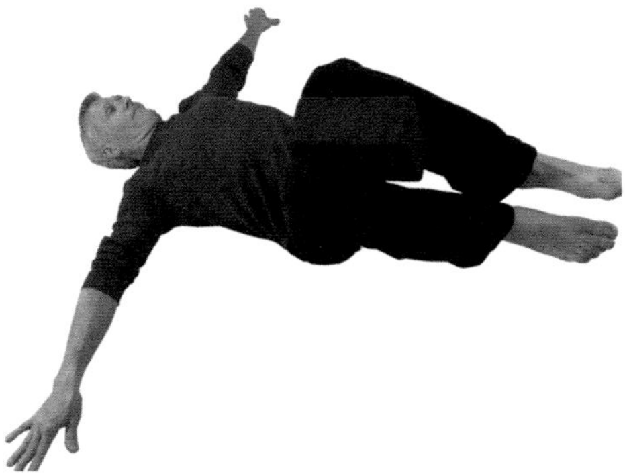

Begin by lying on your back with your knees in toward you and your feet off the floor. Squeeze a yoga block between your thighs (this will help keep your legs moving in harmony), and extend your arms out to a T-shape. From here, draw an infinity symbol (a sideways figure 8) with your knees (both knees move together, in the same direction), turning your head in the opposite direction of your knees as you go. Inhale on one side, exhale on the other. Draw 10 infinity symbols in one direction, then reverse.

BICYCLE

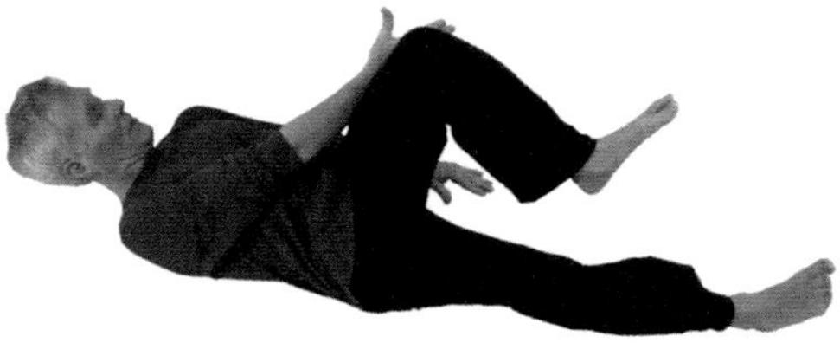

Still supine, remove the block, and bring your forearms to your opposite knees 10 times with your opposite leg extending, like a bicycle (depending on your neck/back strength, your head can lift or stay on the floor). Exhale on the curling effort.

SCISSOR ARMS AND LEGS AND SCISSOR CROSS-PATTERN

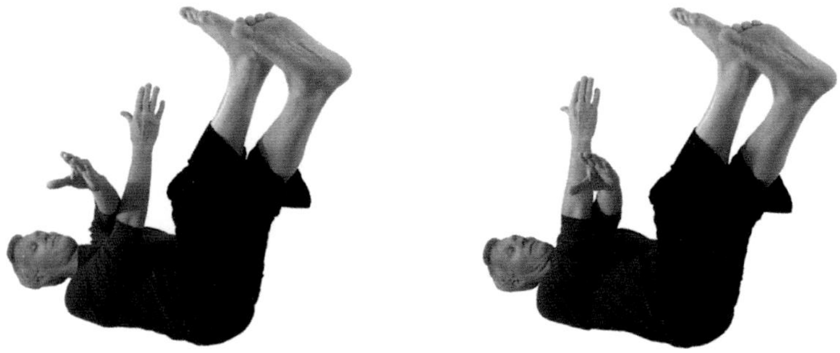

Scissor your arms straight up from your shoulders, then scissor your legs up toward the ceiling as well (your knees can be slightly bent if necessary). Now try scissoring your left arm and right leg on top at the same time. Practice for 1–2 minutes (it's okay to laugh).

STANDING PRACTICE

OPPOSITE ARM ROTATIONS

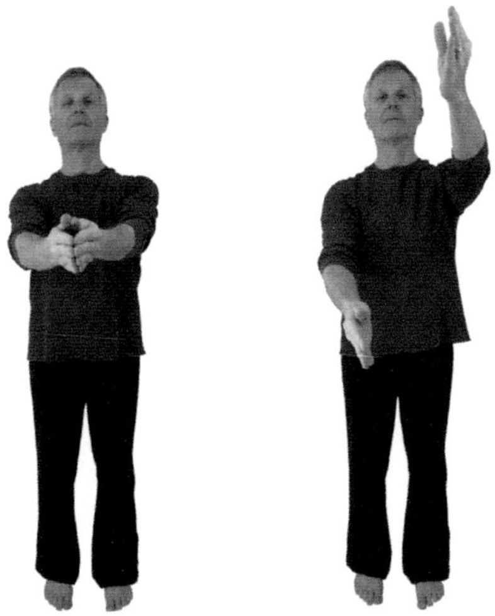

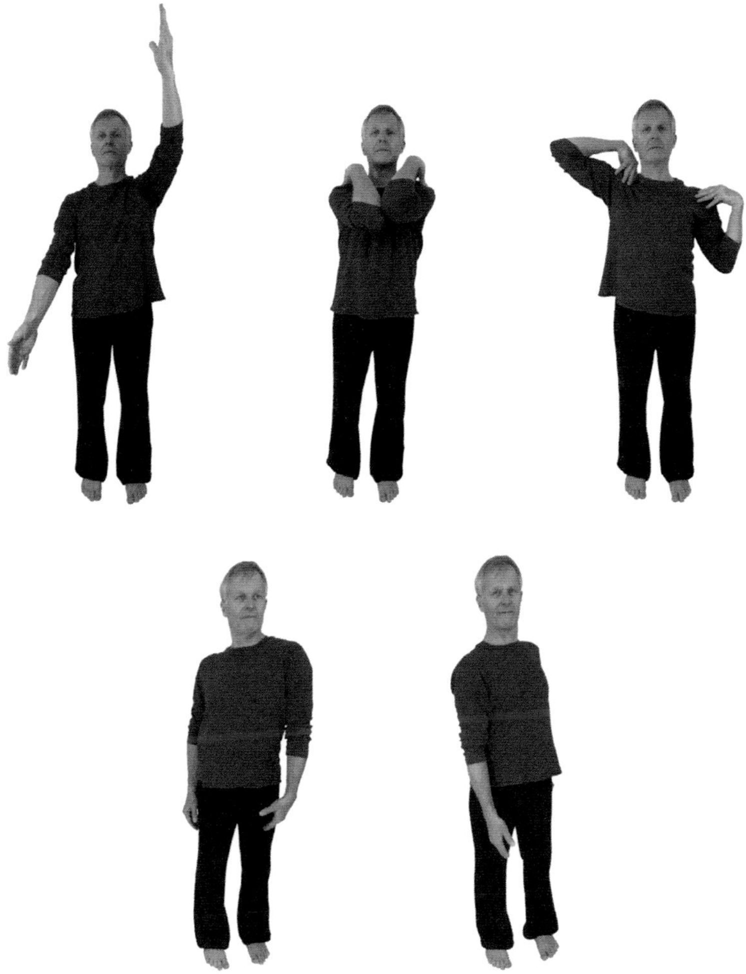

Stand in a stable position, with feet at least hip-distance apart. Open your arms to a wide T (like the first photo in Eagle meets Cow Face Pose on page 140), and then circle your right arm forward and your left arm back. Do this 10 times, and then reverse.

Then do the same thing with your hands resting on your shoulders. Your elbows will touch in front as they come from opposite directions.

The brain will attempt to prohibit the cross-patterning closer to the spinal cord, but try this: Roll one shoulder forward while the other shoulder rolls back about 5 times and then reverse for 5 shoulder rolls. Give yourself lots of room to play with this one.

SLOW STANDING CROSS-CRAWL

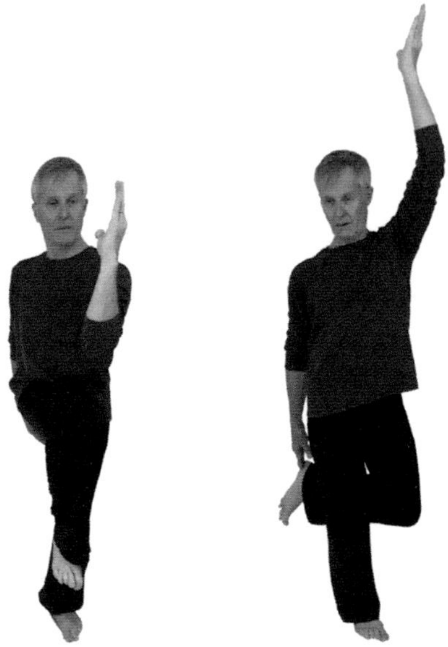

Research has shown that children who have learning disabilities have more difficulty crossing the midline of the body and that earning these skills can help learning as well as improve balance.*

Begin by standing tall with your elbows bent, and slowly lift your right knee up, drawing your left elbow to your right knee, then return to your starting position and switch sides. Take a long, slow exhalation as you draw your knee up to your elbow and an inhalation as you lower back down.

Next, try slowly touching your left heel on an exhalation with your right hand in front of your body, and alternate with touching the opposite heel behind your body. Then alternate elbow to knee, slowly with hand to heel. Trick yourself with new patterns such as front and back on one side, then front and back on the other, then one of each! You're making new neural connections!

* https://childdevelopment.com.au/areas-of-concern/fine-motor-skills/crossing-the-bodys-midline

FIGURE-8 ARMS

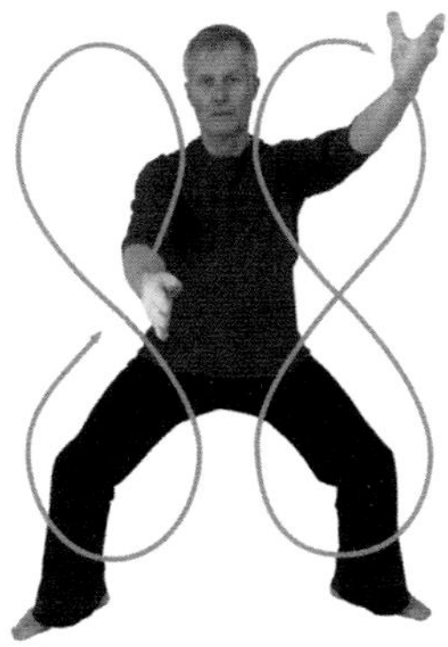

Come into a wide Goddess stance (a high squat). Make forward figure 8s with your arms following the same pattern, then figure 8s in opposite directions, then one figure 8 up and one down. Try as many possibilities as you can.

THOPPUKARANAM (HANDS-TO-EARS *KRIYA*)

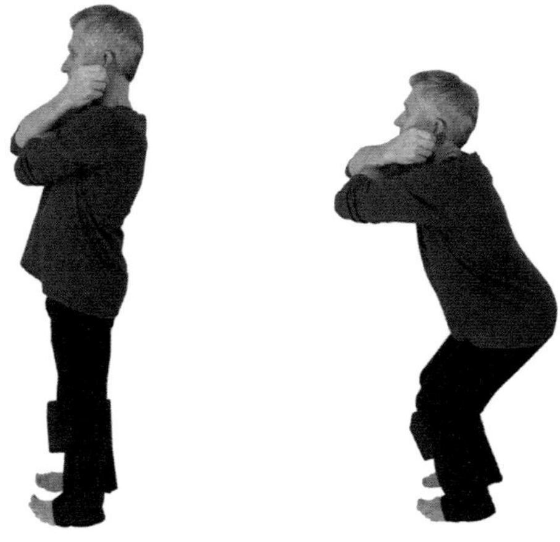

This practice comes from South India and is used in Ganesha temples as an offering of 108 bows. It has also been used in Indian public schools (as punishment for a student not paying attention), but several clinical trials have shown that it helps with mental focus, memory, and mood.[14] You can think of it like "jumper cables" between brain hemispheres as the left hand clasps the right earlobe and the right hand clasps the left earlobe.

Begin in *Tadasana* (Mountain Pose). Bring your left hand to your right earlobe and your right hand to your left earlobe and squeeze gently (in *Ayurvedic* acupuncture this stimulates the pituitary and pineal glands).

Inhale and squat (like you would for Chair Pose), and exhale as you rise, keeping your elbows lifted so you don't round forward.

Begin with 18 squats, inhaling down and exhaling up. Increase your repetitions gradually, working up to as many as 108. When you're finished, I highly recommend you observe how your nostril balance changes. Many students find they have great balance between their left and right nostrils after even a short practice of this *kriya*.

SEATED PRACTICE

EAGLE MEETS COW FACE POSE

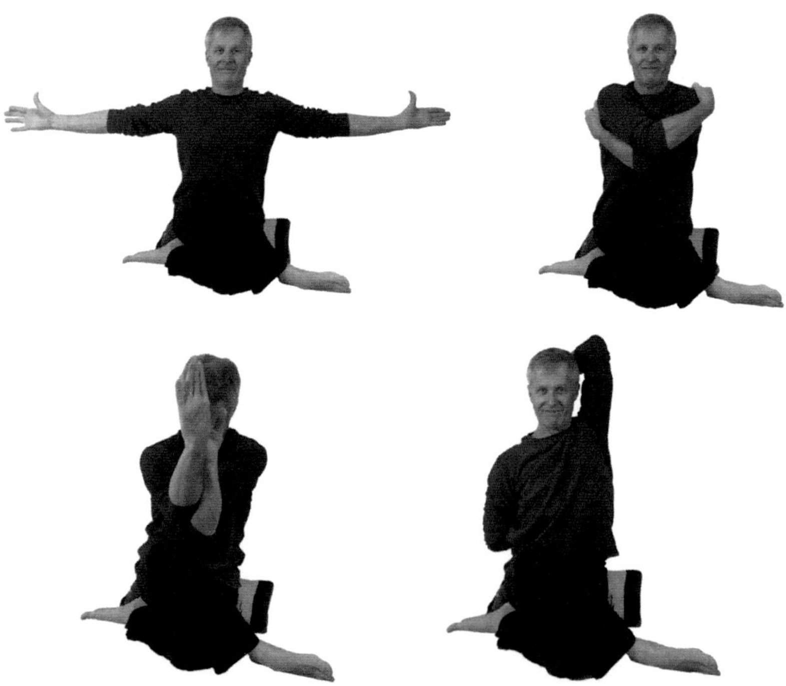

Begin seated on the floor (if your lower back rounds, try elevating your hips on blankets), and cross your right leg over your left— your knees may or may not stack—with your toes pointed back. Open your arms out wide, and hug yourself 3 times, starting with your left arm on top and switching your top arm as you go.

On the third hug, end with your left arm on top (you can place your forearms in Eagle position by weaving them and pressing your lower fingers into the palm of your opposite hand, if you wish). Inhale as you lift your elbows up to chest level and slightly arch your spine. Exhale as you curl inward, drawing your elbows toward your navel. Do this 3 times. Then, unwind your arms, roll out your shoulders, then repeat on the other side.

(Before uncrossing your legs on each side, you could add the classic Cow Face Pose arm position, with your left elbow pointing upward and your right elbow down at the side. Clasp behind your back or reach toward your opposite hand connection with a strap if desired as it gives the shoulders an oppositional stretch, plus it's more cross-patterning!)

SIMPLE SEATED TWIST WITH COUNTERED EYE MOVEMENTS

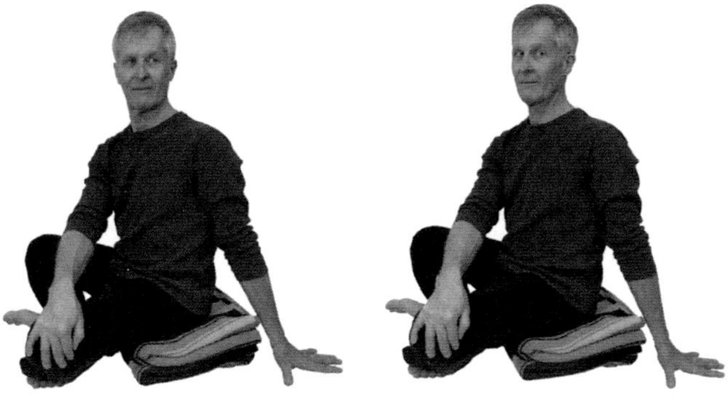

Find a comfortable sitting position, either on a chair or cross-legged on the floor in Easy Posture.

Sit tall, and on an exhale, rotate your torso to the left, turning your head to the left as well. Take your left hand behind you, and put your right hand on your left knee. Then, leave your gaze to the left as you turn your head back toward the right, keeping the breath steady and slow. The movement may feel awkward and jerky, as the nervous system adjusts. Return to face forward slowly and leave your eyes closed a moment. Take your time moving to the other side, then repeat the process to the right. If this procedure makes you feel dizzy, try it as a reclining twist.

Note: Keeping the breath long and deep is very important in this exercise. We often retain our trauma in the patterns of the breath, and resisting holding the breath and doing this movement may be a challenge (especially since at the same time the nervous system and brain are trying very hard to keep the head and eye movement coordinated). This movement is also known as "Releasing the Neck from the Tyranny of the Eyes," so it may help with neck pain as well.

TAKING PICTURES WITH THE EYES

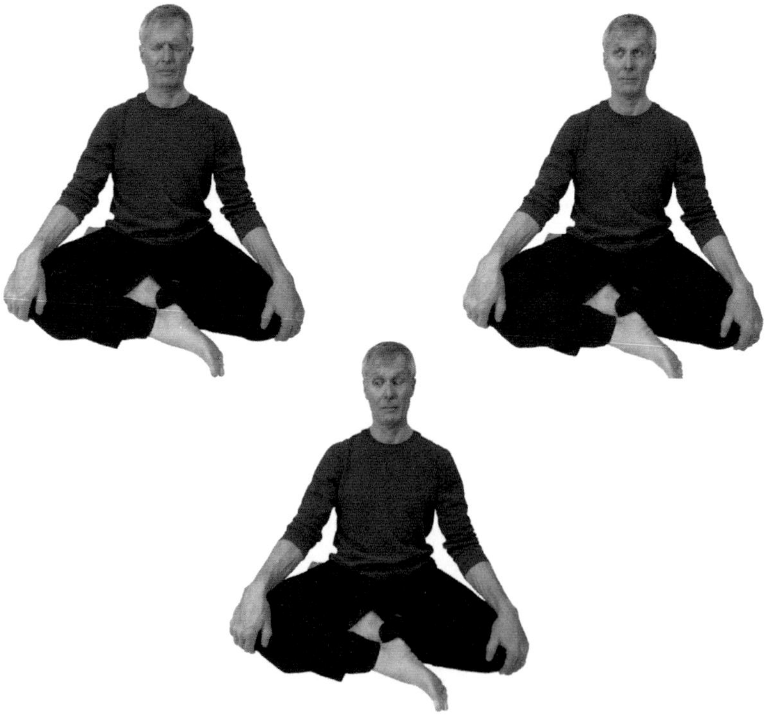

After completing the previous exercise and returning to center, "take pictures" with your eyes. Squeeze them shut and then pop them open at random places in or outside of the room you're in. It may take a minute or more, but snap and pop your eyes open until they feel moist, then rub your hands together and rest your eyes in the darkness of your hands (preferably tilting your head down to rest heavily in your hands) for 5–10 breaths.

Do figure-8 eye exercises in each direction. Loop your eyes to left and right, making horizontal figure 8s, then try reversing the pattern.

The following two exercises are for children or kids at heart!

EARSEY-NOSEY

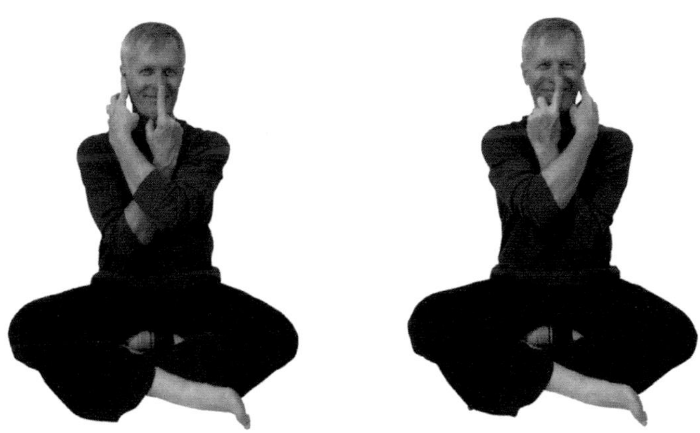

This is a childhood game that involves crossing your wrists and touching an ear on the opposite side of your head with one index finger and your nose with the other, then reversing the crossing of your wrists and doing it on the opposite side. Try 5 rounds. Keep breathing!

FINGER GAME

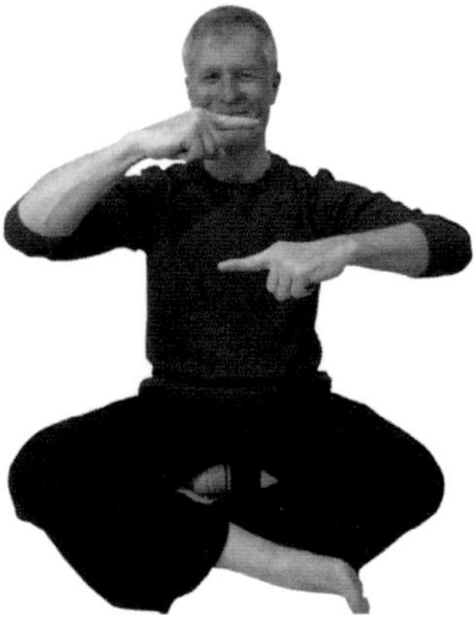

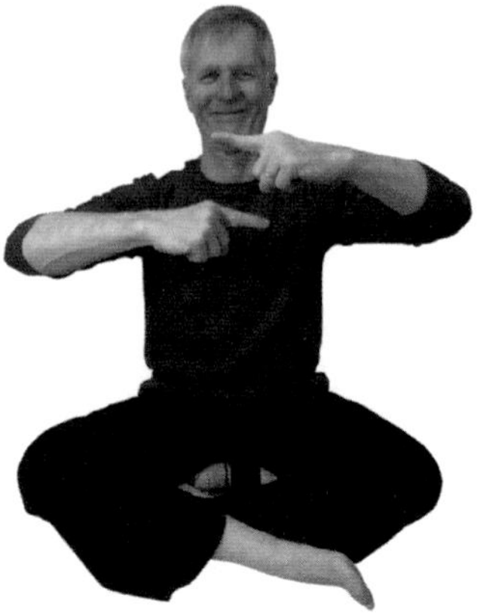

Turn one index finger forward and circle it in the opposite direction with the other index finger. Turn 5–10 times each direction with long deep breaths.

Playground games like "Miss Mary Mack," hopscotch, and pat-a-cake games involve crossing the midline in the body too! If you get a chance to play or teach them to your children or grandchildren, join in! All will benefit.

Have you ever considered how little you cross one side of your body over to the other (unless you are in a yoga class doing twist postures)? Making this circuit is important for our brain health. It helps us to maintain balance and also aids neurological processing. Some people, especially those who have experienced trauma, don't even move their arms in opposition to their legs when walking or running (a natural cross-pattern); they may keep their arms dangling and inert or move the same side as the leg). It is through cross-body movement that our nervous system resets. You won't understand the benefits until you try it. Your brain will thank you.

CHAPTER 8

Fear and the Creative Process

Swadhisthana, *Saraswati* and Fearlessness

Swadhisthana (sacral *chakra*) is located a couple of inches below the navel and near the spine. In writing a book on overcoming fear via Yoga Therapy, it seems odd to me that this piece of the energetic puzzle keeps coming to the fore. Most of us have had our creative endeavors thwarted at some point, often in childhood. Showing our artistic side is like revealing our sacred underbelly; to do so takes great courage. Reconnection with the second or sacral *chakra* is an essential part of moving toward a fuller, less fearful life. Before we delve into this *chakra*, let's first look at the sacrum itself.

The sacrum is the big, heavy, triangular mass of fused bones at the base of the spine. The sacrum is the base on which the vertebrae stack, and one of its main functions is to connect the spine to the hip bones (ilia). Incidentally, it also connects to our tail—yes, we do have one! Our healthy alignment depends on the tilt of the sacrum.

In Yoga Therapy sessions, I often see fear reflected in the posterior tilt and unsteadiness of the sacrum. Just like our furry mammal friends, trauma and abuse are often reflected in tail-tucking behavior. The rest of the spine reflects this rounding as well, as the shoulders roll forward in response. The breath becomes shallower as the chest collapses, and the whole cycle of fear, anxiety, and doubt perpetuates. Our emotions affect our posture, but our posture can also affect our emotions.

The word "sacrum" has Greek and Roman roots, and means "sacred" or "holy." In Greek, the word for sacrum, "*hieron*," also means temple. The sacrum is a temple in the sense that this bony structure protects and houses the ovaries and uterus, the sacred organs of procreation. It is also one of the last bones to decompose after death, and ancients saw it as a piece of the puzzle from which the body could be reassembled in the afterlife. The idea that the sacrum has deeper significance also has origins in Ancient Egypt, where this bone was considered sacred to Osiris, the god of resurrection and of agriculture. We can see from these examples that creativity played a major role in the lore surrounding the sacrum, and creativity is also a key characteristic of the sacral *chakra*. In some yoga traditions, *swadhisthana* is translated as "one's own dwelling place." In the *tantric* traditions I have studied most recently, the translation is "her own dwelling place." Who is the "she" to whom they refer? In the big picture, she is *Kundalini Shakti*, the divine feminine as the potential energy lying dormant in the lower *chakras*; when awakened, she rises up through the *sushumna* (central vertical column) to the higher centers and toward higher consciousness. But she can manifest with many attributes (as the Mother of the Universe would, of course). In the second *chakra* specifically, she is the creative force, the power of sexuality, and our connection to becoming the innovative power we were intended to be.

The second *chakra* is known as the *chakra* of creativity, pure attention, and pure knowledge. It is the switch that triggers inner inspiration and opens the gates to experiencing the beauty around us. It is also believed to be the storage center of past *karmas*. It's not the physical location of the *karmas* that are being healed but the *karmas* that reside in the mind. Awakening energy at the sacral plexus trips the switch so that we can access the means to heal those past *karmas*.

But whether or not you believe in deity energy or *chakras*, here is how this looks on a practical level: When we aren't utilizing our creative gifts—whether because of fear of rejection, lack of confidence, or past abuse—we lose our health in some capacity.

The "flow" process of writing, teaching, gardening, making art, or cooking, which comes from our innate appreciation of beauty or the simple need to be heard, unlocks the repression that keeps us from being fully who we are. This very often shows up in our physical well-being as well as our mental state. Doing and making things we love increases our immune response and gives us a reason to wake up in the morning. Author Nicholas Turiano, now at the University of Rochester Medical Center, said, "Individuals high in creativity maintain the integrity of their neural networks even into old age."[1]

We need to create to be strong, and that strength is reflected in the stability of the pelvis—when the pelvis is off-kilter, it shows up everywhere in the body. I often see a student simultaneously begin to find their artistic side *and* begin to feel more free in the pelvis; or maybe it's just more somatic understanding and connection I see in their sacral/pelvic area.

Many of us wanted to be artists, dancers, or write great books when we were children. These aspirations are especially common at 7–14 years (it's no coincidence that we often have our first crush during this period). Often, something happens during that time that dashes our belief in our creativity. We're told we have no rhythm for dance or no ear for music, the colors we choose are not the same as those favored by the rest of the class, and we despair.

Early humans never questioned being artists;[2] one simply played an instrument, sang, acted out dramatically, or made things, because it is the nature of being human to create. But today many of us have been told it's a waste of time or that we lack talent, so we just stop creating. What a loss. Passion on all levels is affected by lack of creative outlet.

How do we rekindle that quality of delight in "making?" Yoga has methods via *mantra*, *asana*, and movement to help us reconnect with our inner *Saraswati*.

The *bija mantra* (seed sound) for the second *chakra* is "*vam*" and can produce powerful effects on its own when recited or used silently in meditation or within the practice of *Bhuta Shuddhi* (Cleansing of the Elements).* The element for the *swadhisthana chakra* is water, and flow is its nature. Simply chanting or quietly meditating on the *bija vam* can help produce an inner calm; and ultimately, we *like* calming down, though we often fight it in order to feel productive. You may find that chanting it aloud helps bring that quality even more to the forefront of your consciousness.

A *mantra* such as *Om Eim Saraswatyei Swaha* (salutations to that feminine energy which informs all artistic and scholarly endeavors, and for which Eim is the seed), may also appeal to you while envisioning yourself as a part of the creative process.

Gentle work with the breath and pelvic floor can help energize the sacral energy as well. Learning practices such as Root Lock and *Agni Sara* can help us to feel more mobilized in the pelvis; and practicing fewer rigid poses and more dynamic, dance-like, free movement can help us let go of the perfectionism of a structured, alignment-based practice. Moving to music, or your own internal music, is very healing and can help address fear rooted in the body. These freeing actions can be a lovely preparation for moving inward.

Meditation is learning to control the subconscious mind consciously, and one might think it is restrictive to the creative flow. But because of meditation's capacity for lowering anxiety, it can make the gates to our inner artist easier to access. We put aside the drip-drip of our smaller self and become the flow of the ocean. There is so much more that we can express when we have that connection.

So *mantra*, movement, and meditation can help us unlock that blockage and move toward our full expression of our life's purpose.

---

* *Yoga International* has an excellent guide to this practice at https://yogainternational.com/article/view/purify-your-chakras-part-4-how-to-practice-bhuta-shuddhi

MUDRAS TO ADDRESS FEAR

ABHAYA MUDRA (FEAR-DISPELLING *MUDRA*)

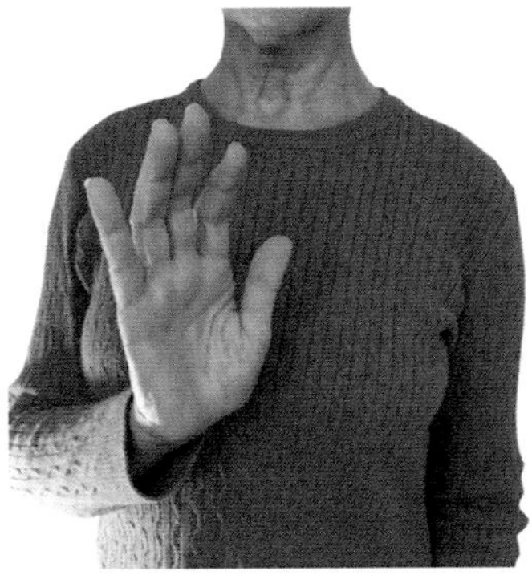

You may have seen statues or representations of sages with the right hand softly facing outward from the heart, radiating peace to the world, allowing the other hand to rest at the side. This is *Abhaya Mudra* and it is a beautiful practice to remind us of that state of being without fear. Hold for 5 minutes breathing slowly and deeply.

HRIDAYA ABHAYA MUDRA (*MUDRA* OF THE FEARLESS HEART)

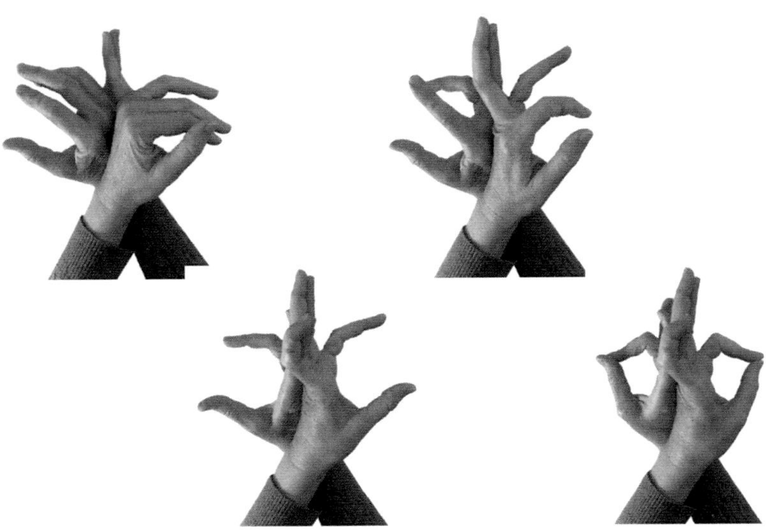

The shape of this *mudra* is reminiscent of a heart with wings, and when held with intention can be quite empowering.

Cross your left wrist in front of your right, then cross the left index finger over the right index finger, the left middle finger over the right middle finger, and the left pinky finger over the right pinky finger (leaving the ring fingers and the thumbs uncrossed). Then touch the tips of the thumbs and the tips of the ring fingers together (right thumb to right ring finger and left thumb to left ring finger) to create the "wings." Position your hands in front of your chest and hold for 5 minutes or longer with long deep breaths.

USING *MANTRA* WITH *MUDRA*

MAHA MRITYUNJAYA (CONQUEROR OF DEATH)

It is said that the *Maha Mrityunjaya Mantra* (Conqueror of Death) was sent by Lord Shiva to destroy the fear of death (*abhinivesha*) and as a tool for healing. Use of the *mantra* is said to restore and rejuvenate. It is also often used before travel, is said to prepare the body to receive medicines more readily, and is recited at the time of death. It's advised to repeat it 3, 11, 21, or 36 times. If using for *japa* (repetition of a *mantra*), a *mala* (a string of 108 beads used for counting repetitions of a prayer or *mantra*, similar to a Catholic rosary) may be used counting rounds of 108.

The Sanskrit text reads:

OM. Tryambakam yajamahe
Sugandhim pushti-vardhanam
Urvarukam iva bandhanan
Mrityormukshiya maamritat

ॐ *aum*—a sacred/mystical syllable in Hinduism, Jainism, Buddhism, and Sikhism

त्र्यम्बकं *tryambakam*—the three-eyed one, Siva

यजामहे *yajmahe*—we worship, adore, honor, revere

सुगन्धिम् *sugandhim*—sweet fragrance, fragrant

पुष्टि *pushti*—a well-nourished condition, thriving, prosperous, fullness of life

वर्धनम् *vardhanam*—one who nourishes, strengthens, causes to increase (in health, wealth, well-being); who gladdens, exhilarates, and restores health; a good gardener

उर्वारुकमिव *urvarukam iva*—like the cucumber or melon

बन्धनान् *bandhanan*—"from captivity" (i.e. from the stem of the cucumber or the gourd)

Note: *bandhanan* means bound down. Thus, read with *urvarukam iva*, it means "I am bound down just like a cucumber (to a vine)." If you read it with *mrtyormukshiya*, it means "liberate from the bounds of death."

मृत्योर्मुक्षीय *mrtyormukshiya*—to free, liberate from death

माऽमृतात् *maamritat*—please give me rejuvenating nectar, so as to have this liberation, like the process of severing the cucumber from the creeping vine

Perhaps the line that perks my interest the most is the one comparing our clinging to life and its suffering to the being bound like a cucumber to the vine, which weaves its tendrils tightly to its support. It reminds me of a story Easwaran would tell us about his grandmother taking him to visit the bedsides of people who were dying, even when he was quite young. He asked her why people cried and wailed so at the time of death. She asked him to sit in a chair and to hold on tightly, and then she yanked him out of the chair. He said she was very strong and it truly hurt. Then she had him sit again, but this time he had to wrap his arms around her neck and allow her to lift him into her arms. He then understood that it is clinging that causes suffering. When taken in regular doses, the *Maha Mrityunjaya Mantra* is said to help ease that clinging.

TRIKHANDA MUDRA (OR *SARVA TRIKHANDA MUDRA*)

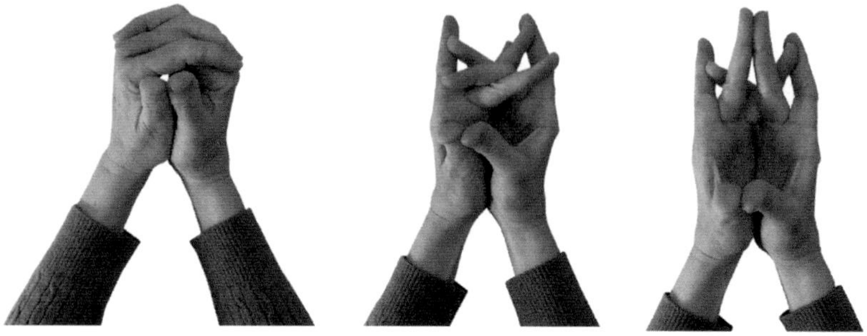

This *mudra* is often combined with *Maha Mrityunjaya Mantra* to act as a "container" or chalice to hold or share the power of the sound. *Trikhanda Mudra* (or *Sarva Trikhanda Mudra*) is beautifully intricate, but in time comes easily. The name "*trikhanda*" suggests the three parts of *Srividya* (meaning highest knowledge, and a major school of *tantric* study) *Mantra*: *Akanda mandalakaram visvam vyaya vyavasthitam trailokya manditam yena mandalam tat sadasivam*. This is known as The *Guru Stotram*, an honorarium to the great teachers, which can be used as an invocation prior to using the *Trikhanda Mudra*, which signifies the principles of the Sun, the Moon, and the Fire (represented by the three ascending fingers on each hand).

This *mudra* is presented by joining and interlacing the fingers of both the hands, but the pinky fingers, middle fingers, and the thumbs point upward and the index is wrapped around the ring finger. The fingers can be unlaced toward you to facilitate personal healing or opened outward toward someone in need of care. Combining *mantra* with *Trikhanda*, which is like a chalice when complete, is like filling the *mudra* with the life force (*prana*) of the living words. Together they create a more powerful healing practice.

CHAPTER 9

I Thought All Yoga Was Therapeutic!

As we were moving slowly and consciously through a series of poses in a Yoga Therapy session last week, a 69-year-old client of mine who had practiced *asana* off and on for 40 years noted the difference between Yoga Therapy and the typical group classes she'd been to in the past, exclaiming, "No wonder I don't attend classes anymore! It doesn't make sense for me to do what they are doing. And I thought all yoga was therapeutic!"

What we came to understand in her session was that many of the poses, instructions, and approaches to fitness that she was encountering in her local yoga classes were aggravating her conditions rather than alleviating them. Was this just because she was no longer 25? Not at all—I've seen the same kind of overuse and repetitive strain in people in their 20s, and even in teenagers. But for some reason, it's a common belief that yoga is exempt from the rules of cross-training and diversity of movement. Students believe they can trust a teacher to keep them safe and are often afraid of not following directions.

Is Fear of Injury in Yoga Class Founded?

Injury has now become so much a part of yoga practice that it is widely accepted as inevitable. I recently came across a Facebook post written by a self-described "yoga teacher/mentor" this week that illustrates this perfectly. Her words (directed to her students) were, to this effect: "We've been through so much together, so many changes. I've seen some of you become mothers, others retire, we've ripped hamstrings, and blown shoulders…" My mouth fell open. Since when are torn hamstrings and injured shoulders a normal, accepted part of the yoga experience? Memorable, yes, but something to look back on with nostalgia? Somehow I don't think that sages of yoga would agree, since yogis ascribe to the same rule of *ahimsa* (the principle of non-violence) as do medical doctors—first, do no harm.

More and more, doctors are offering referrals to yoga classes, and teachers and students alike must be aware of what that means. Within the medical community, there is a growing sense of trust in yoga and in yoga teachers. My classes at a hospital, and my private lessons and therapy sessions, were full of doctors, nurses, physical and occupational therapists, and their families. Many of these medical professionals even chose to go through yoga teacher training programs so that they would have new options to offer their patients.

The issue is that, to most people, a "yoga class" means "follow the leader," and includes the same 20 or so poses in every class. Some of them might feel good, like the reclining bent-knee-over-straight-leg twist that makes your back pop every time. This type of twist is actually destabilizing for your lumbar joints and, when done repeatedly, may lead to arthritis or sciatic nerve issues. Is it really worth it? And while it may be momentarily empowering to kick up into Headstand so you can say, "I nailed that pose," what about the nagging nail of a neck pain the next morning? Or maybe you love the achievement of Full Lotus but are noticing knee pain. Thankfully, there are other poses out there—poses that may make you stronger and more flexible. But discovering those poses takes time and demands attention to the specific needs of your body.

To see why a "one-size-fits-all" approach to yoga can be problematic, let's look at the outline of a standard yoga class. It starts with some kind of warm-up. This, in my opinion, is the most important part of the class. Exploring the body's tightness *du jour*, using breath to find supple ease for the day or de-stressing in the evening is why most students say they come to class. If left to our own devices, many of us might choose to spend anywhere from 20 minutes to an entire class doing Cat/Cow variations and all the core work and delicious hamstring and shoulder stretches we want. But before we know it, we are up and into Sun Salutes (or a comparable *vinyasa*) because the fitness class model demands that unless we sweat we aren't "doing yoga."

In my private work, more than three-quarters of my diverse clientele are unable to benefit their current physical state very much by doing "Sun Salutes" as they know them. Their backs are rounded in Forward Folds, their knees locked in Downward Dog, and their heads flung back as they grasp for Backbends by straining upward; a *Chaturanga* is a belly flop with shoulders wailing in misery, and stepping forward from Downward Dog is an arduous and pretty embarrassing process. Many of my clients hate these Sun Salutes but have done them religiously—thinking they were required in yoga practice and therefore must be good for them. With new or untrained teachers especially, Sun Salutes often take up a good amount of class time as they may not be aware of other ways to generate heat.

Next come standing poses. Despite the fact that even students who have practiced for years have alignment epiphanies when they raise the surface at which they practice, in an average class, modifications with a chair or other high surfaces are almost never offered for standing postures such as Triangle. (If the agile teacher and the other students are using no props, it could be embarrassing to pull out a chair—especially if the student is young, or older but wanting to appear strong and healthy. This is another instance of a difference between a therapeutic and a generalized fitness approach that we'll explore more on page 161.)

After a few standing poses, many yoga classes include some sort of inversion—often much too difficult for those lacking core and arm strength. More experienced teachers will give some helpful modifications, since falling out of an upside-down pose can be pretty scary (as are lawsuits). Poses such as Legs Up the Wall or Legs Up a Chair are wonderful, accessible inversions. And for those with more arm strength, a Handstand or Forearm Balance is actually less risky than a Headstand or unsupported neck-smashing Shoulder Stand. But even so, practitioners often eschew the simple poses in favor of more dramatic or "classical" postures. While inversions can be very beneficial for the body and mood, keeping your head and neck safe is an essential part of the practice!

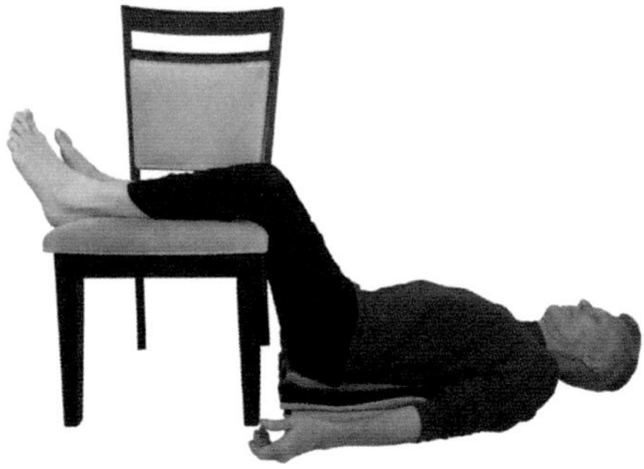

Figure 8.1 Legs Up a Chair Pose

The backbending part of class is excellent for many people, and a well-aligned Bridge or Locust can be quite strengthening. But when the other students start jamming stiff arms into full Cobras, or teachers lift students into full Wheels so that everyone "gets there," many practitioners feel pressured to do things for which their own bodies will suffer (both now and later).

Twists can be the most subtle and luscious of *asanas* when approached in an informed and exploratory fashion. But a "get it done" mentality takes much of the sweetness out of the twist. Going for a popping "adjustment" or squeezing excessively to "wring out toxins" promotes an aggressive approach to the spinal movement. In actuality, it is the breath that promotes the "detox," not the twists "flushing the organs with new blood." Of course, gentle twisting can help to calm the nervous system and keep the spine mobile. Popping is not always a good thing, though, and may set you up for joint problems down the line.

In many classes, there tends to be a similar approach to Forward Folds, which should be calming, soothing, strengthening, and lengthening poses. The "If you are more flexible, do…" cue becomes a punishment to those whose natural suppleness (or lack thereof) may not meet their own expectations. They begin pulling and tugging themselves forward with rounded lumbar spines. When you consider the sitting that most of us do all day, why would collapsing and squeezing our spinal discs be a good plan?

Along the same lines, you'll probably also find the ubiquitous "Hip Openers" in most classes. These are beneficial to a degree and may feel good to tightly clenched buttocks—but when over-practiced without good core strength and a countering squeeze from the outer thighs, they can cause instability of the hip joint. My motto is "Don't feed the pigeon," especially if it's a fat, spacious pigeon with way too much entitlement. In other words, if the pose feels too easy, the student needs to strengthen the muscles around the joint rather than increase a passive stretch. Loosen what's too tight, tighten what's too loose.

Along with warm-ups, *Savasana* relaxation has the opportunity to be a particularly healing part of the yoga class, especially when attention is given to diaphragmatic breathing. In fact, some really great teachers add a sprinkling of "stop, breathe, and pay attention" practice throughout their classes, or start class with a centering resting pose. It is in the moments of resting that our minds and bodies download what we have practiced. Without the stopping and resting, the autonomic nervous system can't assimilate the deeper benefits. Conscious rest provides a training ground for keeping us calm in all of life's stressful situations.

What I'm talking about is yoga as a healing modality—not just for weight loss or "detox," or to firm buttocks or perform impressive postures. I had one Yoga Therapy client who really understood the difference. She said, "I am here for the therapy, the process that happens in the breath and mind and body. I also do fitness yoga, a vigorous power flow, because I don't like running!" She practiced yoga as therapy, along with yoga as fitness, and did not confuse the two.

If a healthy person with a clear mind and good joints and muscles takes vigorous classes to stay fit, good for them! But they need to vary their movements and be aware of the pitfalls of some repetitive actions too. RSI or repetitive strain injury can be caused by repeated or continual movement, such as vibrations, awkward positions that are prolonged or mechanical compression, and can cause damage to the nervous system and musculo-skeletal system. How many awkward positions do we assume repeatedly in yoga classes, especially in *vinyasa*? (Think weight supported on hands, neck thrust back.) How many times per week? Or if you are a teacher, how many times per day?

If you are unsure about how to practice therapeutically, it may be good to visit a well-recommended Yoga Therapist or experienced teacher who can map out some areas where you need strength practices, and others where you need to focus on flexibility. Consulting with the International Association of Yoga Therapists (IAYT) for trained therapists in your area may be helpful. Most importantly, a trained professional can observe how you breathe during yoga and help you to modify the speed and intensity of your practice accordingly. This type of help will give the prospective or long-term yogi more confidence in how to practice in general. Remember: The poses and breathing techniques we choose to practice may lower pain levels and help with range of motion, but it's *how* we practice them that can change our lives.

I'm not offering these thoughts to frighten students or keep them away from classes they love. But how many times must we ignore the pinches we feel around the tops of our thighbones, or the lower back twinges in straight-leg Forward Folds? How many times must we continue to lower to *Chaturanga* when it hurts our shoulders? When we "do it anyway" (just like going for a third cocktail or chocolate pie bender), we will pay for it sooner or later.

If you attend classes because you love them, consider trying the simpler "beginner's" options for a while. Go on your knees in Plank Pose, or skip the deep backbends even if you think you can do them—then gradually add other moves/positions from there. Ask yourself: Is this uncomfortable? Is my breath ragged? Am I stressed or anxious when I try this? If a teacher pushes you to ever-harder movements that result in pain, or won't let you modify a pose, look for a new class.

My personal preference is to let my yoga be sweet yoga, and take a long walk (with attention to alignment!) if I want fitness. My "sweet" practice includes different strong *asana* every day, along with plenty of TLC. My body has been at this awhile and rewires well with some intense focused poses. This may be the case for you as well.

The home remedy I suggest for anyone is to be more playful in your practice—to breathe and stretch in joyful ways that generate a sense of openness in your body. Historically, before the development of *asana* as we know it, yogis simply moved to link the circuits in their energetic systems. They would then "breathe life" into these shapes. In fact, *Tandava* (Indian sacred dance) and *Qigong* both evolved out of playful, wise, joyful movement combined with breath.

Start on the floor on your belly or back and just see what your breath is doing; then move your way into cat-like stretches—not necessarily a yoga pose, but stretching to feel better and to connect with deeper breathing into tight areas. And when you discover the yoga postures that give you space, allow you to breathe deeper "into" constricted areas of your body, and leave you feeling refreshed, practice them! Practice them in a spirit of exploration.

Swami Rama of the Himalayas, a spiritual scientist and remarkable scholar of the mind/body connection, likewise encouraged his students to be like scientists in exploring the body and energetic system. But no good laboratory research is done without variables or by allowing oneself to damage the equipment. Explore and learn your strengths and weaknesses, and vary what you are doing physically. Only a mad scientist does the same thing over and over and expects a different result.

Yoga Therapy versus Yoga Class

I've offered Yoga Therapy for 25 years. I've also taught both gentle and vigorous *Hatha* Yoga in various styles for over 40 years in education centers, studios, fitness centers, and hospitals. Through it all, I've learned a lot about the nature of Yoga Therapy—namely, that there is a difference between classroom *asana* and Yoga Therapy. Teaching in a classroom setting, I became aware that students come to their mats with every conceivable physical and emotional quandary. Generalized safe movement and breath practices may help to address some of these, but more focused time spent looking at how all the pieces of yoga fit with attention to individual needs provides deeper and more direct benefits.

When scheduling private therapy sessions, people often assume they will receive the same set of practices that are offered in a gentle yoga class. Yoga Therapists, however, are not simply teachers or personal trainers, but rather trained therapists offering specific techniques in breath, physical movement, sound, and sometimes *mudras* and meditation practices to assist healing. Yoga Therapists look at how you walk, sit, and stand—and even how you eat—helping you create healthy new patterns and allowing you to take charge of your own well-being.

Below are some common assumptions (and clarifications) to assist in differentiating between yoga classes and Yoga Therapy.

Assumption #1: People must be able to get up from the floor and lower down to the floor to practice yoga

Mobility issues often prevent people from attending yoga classes. Knee, hip, and lower back problems may make lowering to the floor painful and embarrassing. An injured or weak shoulder or wrist can also make getting up from the floor challenging. A class that requires students to lower their bodies to the floor may keep an individual from returning, even if the class is truly needed. Private Yoga Therapy can help a client assess their abilities and limitations in a setting free from rush or embarrassment.

Of course, there are chair-yoga classes. I love them, and I love to teach them—but not everyone can attend these classes, as they may be offered at inconvenient times or in inaccessible locations.

Teachers for such classes are less likely to be available because yoga teacher training often doesn't offer components for instructing those with mobility issues. Chair-assisted classes are also often held during work or school hours and seem intended for those who are retired. As a result, even when chair yoga is available, younger students may feel self-conscious about attending classes marketed toward an older crowd, and students of all ages often have the misconception that chair-based yoga is not "real yoga."

A Yoga Therapist can help make the call about whether chair yoga or other types of practice will benefit the student, and how yoga can be adapted for home practice. A Yoga Therapist focuses on healing rather than specific poses or positions, understanding that there are all kinds of ways to accomplish that end. While a student may want to be able to get up and down off the floor easily, the therapist recognizes that it may not be a rapid process after injury or surgery. If fielded into an all-levels class (even one offering modifications), the student may feel a need to push too hard when seeing others practice. Even in private yoga sessions, many teachers without therapeutic training may assume that a student is there to gain access to harder yoga poses rather than find ease in daily movement.

Assumption #2: We must start and end each class by closing our eyes and centering

Having worked in trauma therapy for many years, I have seen the discomfort created for some students who are expected to close their eyes or lie face down in a yoga practice—for example, often in a yoga class the teacher makes suggestions like starting in Child's Pose or Crocodile Pose, which may serve the majority of students but can cause physical or mental stress for others. Traumatized individuals often exhibit hypervigilance, maintaining an abnormal awareness of environmental stimuli. This can lead to great stress when they are asked to "relax" or "surrender" (even outside of a group setting).

As happens in Zen meditation practices, we can learn to breathe and center with our eyes open, and therapists and some classroom teachers offer this as an option. Yoga Therapy allows for more of an alliance between the therapist and practitioner, creating a conversation about readiness: It is up to the client to decide if and when they are ready to rest their eyes in relaxation or centering.

Assumption #3: Young people need a vigorous class and don't have health issues

We all experience illness and dysfunction at different points in our lives. For some, it may be in youth. Younger students often feel pushed to achieve athletic and even gymnastic feats when practicing anything with the "yoga" label attached. Injuries, disorders, and emotional and mental disturbances are not uncommon in younger students, but young people are often quite uncomfortable coming to a "gentle" yoga class filled with students many years their senior. For these individuals, private Yoga Therapy may be a more comfortable option after (for example) a sports injury or car accident, and it gives young people without current illnesses or injuries the opportunity to deal with individual concerns and develop personal strategies for wellness. This could include tutorials on specific yoga postures that may benefit their healing, or alternatives for practices that need to be avoided or modified.

I've also taught many therapeutically focused group classes to individuals in their teens and 20s. In these types of classes, a Yoga Therapist with additional training in mental and behavioral health issues, or a psychotherapist with yoga training, assists participants in addressing addiction, depression, trauma, or eating disorders, and utilizes breathing and movement specifically designed to help.

Young people are no less vulnerable to the difficulties of life, and we all need nurturance, understanding, and an occasional boost. Yoga Therapy can address complex issues at many levels—physical, hormonal, emotional, mental, and spiritual—and may help in identifying a common thread between a physical issue (e.g. back pain), and how that relates to emotional stressors (e.g. school worries or lack of self-confidence).

Assumption #4: Slow means gentle, and gentle means therapeutic

I was not available one week to lead the Yoga Therapy class in the hospital in which I practiced, and another yoga teacher was sent in to work with a group of orthopedic patients, many of whom had knee and hip replacements or spinal fusions. The teacher offered a regular fitness-focused yoga class but at a very slow pace. Anyone who has held a balance pose or a Warrior stance for over a minute would recognize this as a bigger challenge than a short hold. Needless to say, the hospital staff heard many complaints. Fortunately, no one was hurt, as these long-term students knew their capabilities and modified their movements accordingly.

Is all of Yoga Therapy slow-paced? Not at all. There are times when vigor is helpful, especially when dealing with certain types of depression, addiction, breathing issues, edema, and anxiety. It is case by case. There is no set pace, but Yoga Therapy is always mindful.

Assumption #5: You can assess a student's level of ability and mobility by watching them walk into the class

Years spent in the fields of yoga and Yoga Therapy mean years spent observing people. If I see a person who is thin, young, dressed in athletic wear, with no limp or external indicators of pain, I still cannot assume that they can move comfortably. I have also been surprised at the overall easy movement of people with visible evidence of disability or injury.

At the start of a class, many good teachers ask their students if there are health issues to be considered. Even then, students may not inform the teacher of a personal problem due to embarrassment or limited time before class, hoping to "do what they can." In private Yoga Therapy, clients are more likely to open up about injuries, surgeries, and chronic conditions, and can expect the therapist to offer a broad array of healing possibilities beyond conventional poses.

There are also times when even the most fit among us may find themselves injured or immobilized by a life event. In a group yoga class, it's beyond the teacher's scope of practice to root out trauma or shame, and it would be insensitive to attempt to do so. That is a private matter.

A yoga class—even a gentle yoga class—is not a therapy session. This is not to say that a yoga class is without therapeutic value, and many people may not ever need a one-to-one Yoga Therapy session to better their health. But Yoga Therapy addresses issues that traditional group classes cannot. Yoga therapy is an invaluable way of learning to bring healing to where we personally need it most.

CHAPTER 10

Guts! Yoga and Digestive Health

Michael D. Gershon, an expert in anatomy and cell biology at Columbia University and author of the bestseller *The Second Brain*, states:

> We know that…the gastrointestinal system is equipped with a brain. The unpleasant bowel is more intellectual than the heart and could have a superior "emotional" capacity. It is the only organ to contain an intrinsic nervous system capable of mediating the reflections in the complete absence of input from brain or spinal cord.[1]

He follows up this gusty statement by saying:

> Just think that the gut, while having only a tenth of the neurons of the brain, working independently, helps to fix the memories related to emotions and plays a key role in signaling joy and pain. In short, the intestine is the site of a second brain itself. It is no coincidence the gut cells produce 95% of serotonin, the neurotransmitter of well-being.[2]

For most of us, old mental and emotional patterns keep doing the same things repeatedly and this communication goes right to our gastrointestinal tract. Our good microbes take a hike in the inclement climate of stress and poor eating and the message that we are in a state of emergency—that we are full of distress and disease—is sent to our brains and every single cell in the body.

The goal of Yoga Therapists and our *Ayurvedic* allies is to put out this fire and reassure the lymphatic mind/gut[3] that we are okay and can continue with the good life to which we are entitled.

Gut health is a cultural (no pun intended) rock star right now, as well it should be. How well we digest underlies the smooth function of every system in the body. But is it just about what we eat? If we are trying to digest in a stressed-out body and mind, the benefits of all those great antioxidants and proenzymes may not have as much impact as we'd like. Adding a regular (2–3 times per week) yoga practice to our regimen can impact gut health in a measurable way.

If you or your students are interested in weight management, be aware that a more vigorous type of practice might be necessary to burn calories (though one study[4] showed that overweight women with diabetes lost weight doing Restorative Yoga!). However, a calming practice can improve your body's rhythms, your ability to digest and detoxify, and may even help with depression and low energy levels. We all know that our health, weight, and appetite are deeply affected by mood swings, and practicing yoga is an intelligent and often enjoyable way to address depression and anxiety.

It is important to remember that digestive issues are real and often painful and distressing. They cannot be dismissed as "just my mind working overtime." Anyone diagnosed with Crohn's disease, ulcerative colitis, or other serious digestive problems, should check with their doctor before starting a practice. Letting the yoga teacher or therapist know about a diagnosis can help to avoid any practices that might not be best for a condition. Yoga can be highly beneficial for people who suffer from these chronic conditions, but anyone recovering from an obstruction or surgery should make sure their body is ready to practice. In cases of chronic acid reflux (GERD)[5] and for irritable bowel syndrome (IBS)[6] there is great evidence for yoga's benefit.

Underlying yoga's benefit for digestive ailments is the stimulation of vagal nerve tone.[7] Our old friend the vagus nerve connects to all major organs (including the stomach) and encourages healthy, optimal function of the digestive tract so all the systems of the body work together in a more unified way.

Sounds like a winning plan, but where to begin?

As with any physical regimen, beginning gently is wise—breath-centered Restorative Yoga should be a safe bet, but it may not be necessary to wait for all bowel irregularity or stomach aches to subside to begin a more vigorous practice. Remember that asking a doctor is always a good idea. Recommend your students to start their beginning or "gentle" yoga class in a non-heated studio, as heat can aggravate inflammation. Classes that emphasize deep, relaxed breathing will help promote the relaxation response, which can help us become more mindful in our eating and daily life. If our belly is happier, we'll be happier and much more likely to make the choices that keep our digestive tract on track.

Know that all changes don't happen immediately, and we may need several weeks to notice subtle differences. Self-care isn't a pill we can pop, but the time it takes will be worth it because our daily *sadhana* is a regimen we can use for life with no negative side effects.

Below are some yoga postures and practices to promote digestive health, followed by a simple restorative sequence to practice afterwards or on its own. The chapter ends with a *mudra* for digestion.

A PRACTICE TO PROMOTE DIGESTIVE HEALTH

BALASANA (CHILD'S POSE)

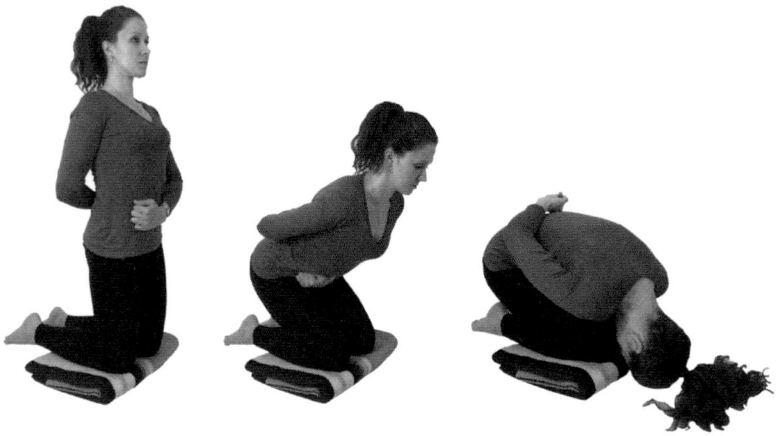

Inhale as you kneel upright with your right forearm behind your back, and exhale as you wrap your ribs over your left arm, with your soft left fist held to your right abdomen. Do this once on each side for 5–10 breaths.

CAT/COW

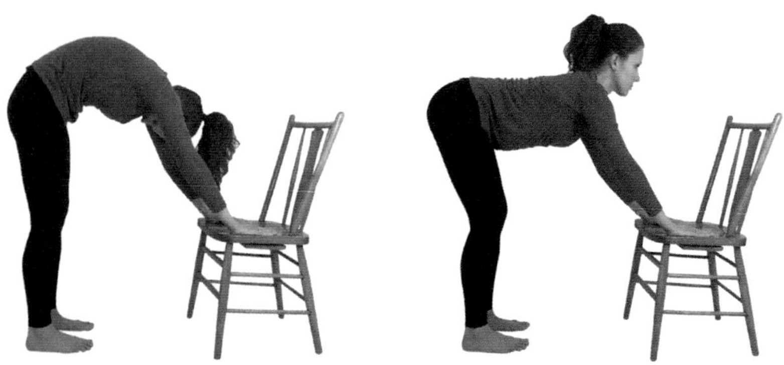

Stand in front of the seat of a chair (standing with your hands on the chair will offer more stimulation to the part of the stomach meridian that extends down your leg). Exhale deeply as you "dome" your spine into the Cat, and inhale as you straighten into the Cow. Do 10 rounds.

PLANK

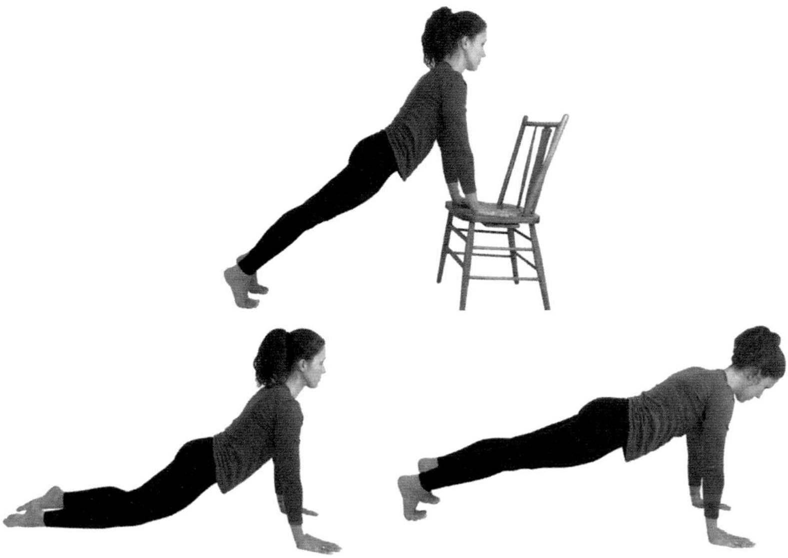

You can do the Plank with a chair or on the floor. To move into Plank, place your hands securely on the outer edges of the chair seat and step back until your feet align diagonally with your head and shoulders. If there are issues with your shoulders or wrists, your Plank may be angled a little at the hip. For a "full Plank," your straight arms support your whole body as you firm your core muscles. For a "half Plank," your knees and lower legs remain on the floor. Stay for 5 breaths.

AGNI SARA (ABDOMINAL SQUEEZE)

There are many ways to practice *Agni Sara*:

Version 1

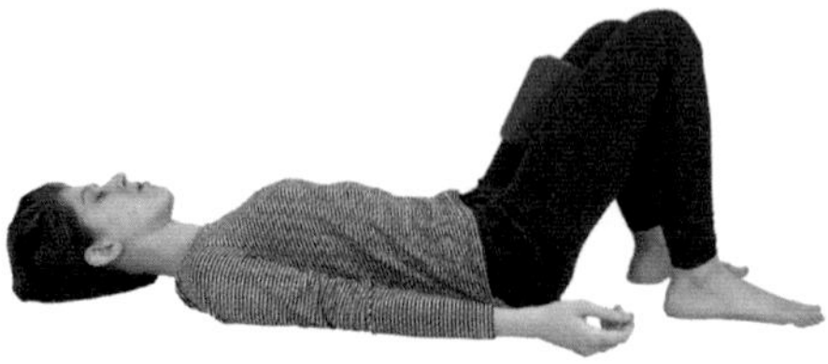

Lie on your back with a block between your thighs, knees bent, and feet flat on the floor. Inhale and as you exhale, engage your pelvic floor. Gradually, in successive breaths, move the contraction to your lower abdomen and (if you have no reflux or ulcer issues) gradually and smoothly contract your upper belly as well. It is good to start with 10 rounds.

Version 2

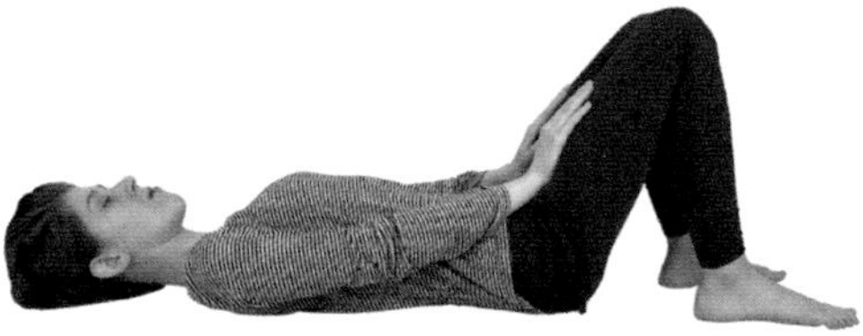

Lie on your back with your knees bent and feet flat on the floor. Place your hands on the tops of your thighs, with your fingers pointing toward your knees. Inhale, then on an exhalation, engage your pelvic floor, lower belly, and upper belly. Suspend (hold out) your exhalation and hollow out your lower belly as if you're "vacuum packing" it up into your upper belly. If you don't have any gastro-intestinal issues, take it higher, sucking your upper belly up under your ribcage. Then, on an inhalation, release your upper belly, lower belly, and pelvic floor, returning to your starting position. The repetitions may be gradually increased over time from 5 to 20.

Version 3

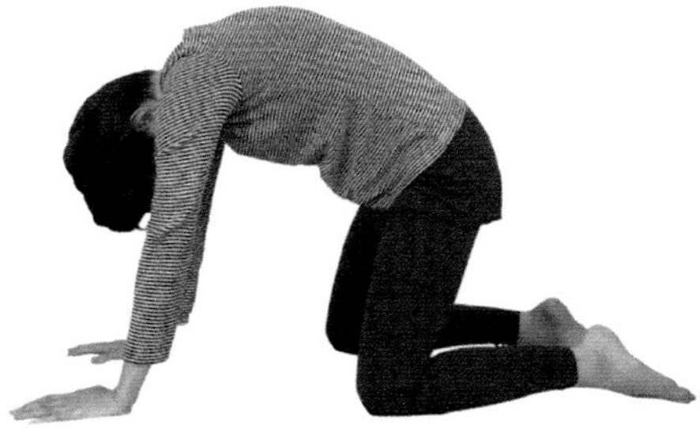

You can also practice *Agni Sara* in Table Position (all fours), or standing with your hands on the seat of a chair. Use the same technique as above. Focus on the abdominal contractions on exhalations at an appropriate depth for your condition (as you did reclining). The repetitions may be gradually increased over time from 5 to 20.

Version 4

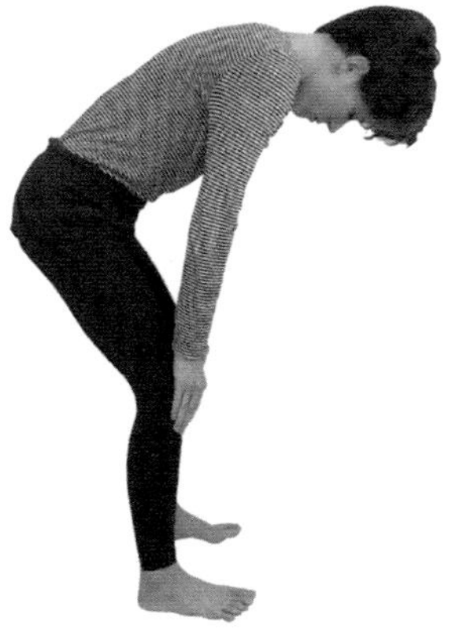

For the "classic" *Agni Sara*, stand with your feet a little wider than hip-width apart, and your hands above your bent knees. Exhale with pelvic floor and abdominal contractions, fully allowing the inhalations to relax your abdominals but keeping some tone in your pelvic floor. Start with 10 rounds and build your practice to 5 minutes.

See what these practices do for you and then if you're a teacher or therapist, look at what's appropriate for the client or student standing in front of you. How much can they apply and understand? I'm often surprised by how clients—even those with no yoga experience—respond to the subtlest of cues.

RESTORE YOUR DIGESTIVE HEALTH: AN EASY RESTORATIVE PRACTICE

The following short restorative practice is for those who feel they need to push ever further into making yoga a challenging workout. It only takes 6 minutes and it can fit nicely at the end of an active yoga sequence.

This practice requires minimal props! You can do the sequence with just a bolster or even a couple of blankets folded into bolster-length rectangles and stacked on top of each other.

Many *pittic* types are often subject to gut issues, especially acid reflux, ulcers, and IBS. Allowing them to understand that they can accomplish something as they relax can help the gut/brain connection. The sensitive digestive system responds well to relaxation techniques.[8]

This is an example of what I might say to someone who really doesn't like to relax:

> I get it, you like to feel strong and accomplished at the end of your yoga practice. You enjoy a good sweat, and Restorative Yoga may seem too boring. Maybe you find it hard enough to remain still through *Savasana* at the end of your *vinyasa* class. So why on earth would you want to spend an entire practice in simple, supported poses?
>
> Let me try to persuade you.
>
> Perhaps you'd like to reap some of restorative yoga's benefits, such as balancing the neuroendocrine system,

> boosting immunity, gut health, weight loss (surprise!), and even increasing compassion for ourselves and others.
>
> The deep relaxation of a restorative practice is also a wonderful complement for the fitness aspects of yoga.
>
> And it can help you access yoga's subtler benefits—such as deepening the breath, relaxing the muscles, and stimulating the vagus nerve and its connection between organs and the brain through supported work—which can balance out the vigor that's integral to a more active practice.

We might ask those who shy away from quiet and stillness to try the following restorative sequence and see if it would be useful with "fierier" constitutions. It is designed especially for those who aren't particularly fond of Restorative Yoga, or for anyone who may just be hesitant to give it a try. You may see relaxation as lazy, but it is a learned skill that helps you be more productive in time. For this sequence more props can always be added to enhance comfort for, in truth, being uncomfortable doesn't earn us any points.

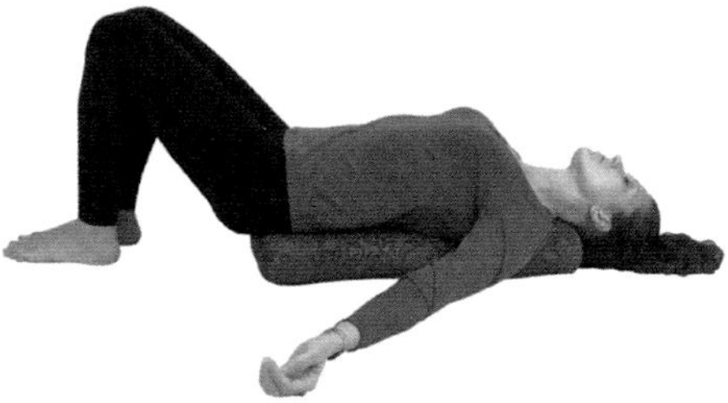

Place the bolster or blanket stack lengthwise on your mat. Sit on the bottom edge of the bolster and lie back so that your head drapes over the top edge (it will rest at about the middle of your neck) with your chin pointing up.

If your head doesn't touch the floor and your neck is uncomfortable with your head dangling, place a folded blanket underneath your head for support.

Bend your knees so that your feet are on the floor (it might feel good to widen your stance and allow your knees to relax in toward each other), and let your arms relax alongside the bolster, with palms facing up (you can also prop your lower legs on the seat of a couch or cushy chair, if you like).

Deepen your breath, allowing your abdomen to rise and fall, and let the muscles of your neck and throat soften. Stay here for 2 minutes.

Next, slide back about 6 inches so that the top of the bolster is now at the middle of your shoulder blades, and your upper back, shoulders, and head are resting on the floor.

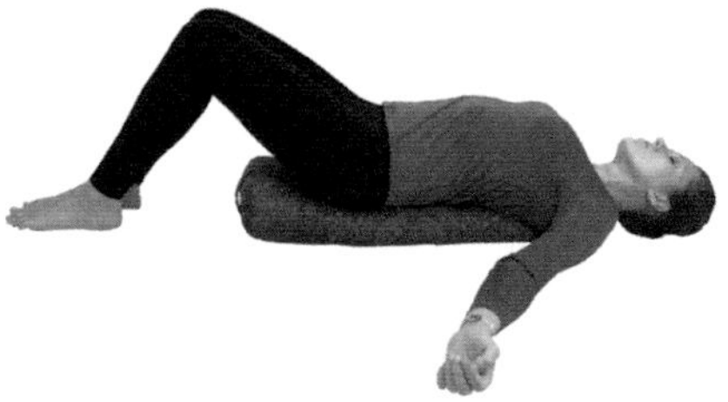

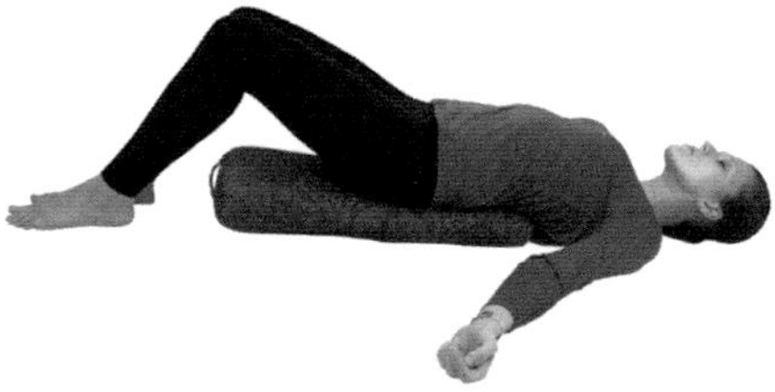

Allow your arms to remain relaxed at your sides. If your legs are on a sofa or chair, you can keep them there; or if it's more comfortable, place your feet on the floor (feet and knees about hip-width apart for this variation).

As you breathe, let your chest and belly expand. For the next 2 minutes, focus on deepening and lengthening your exhalations and letting tension ease in your upper back.

Then, slither back another 6 inches or so until the top edge of the bolster is now below your ribcage. Keep your feet either propped up or on the floor with your arms at your sides. Let your breath expand from your abdomen to your chest for another 2 minutes, noticing the softness of your entire back (and perhaps a bit less resistance to gravity).

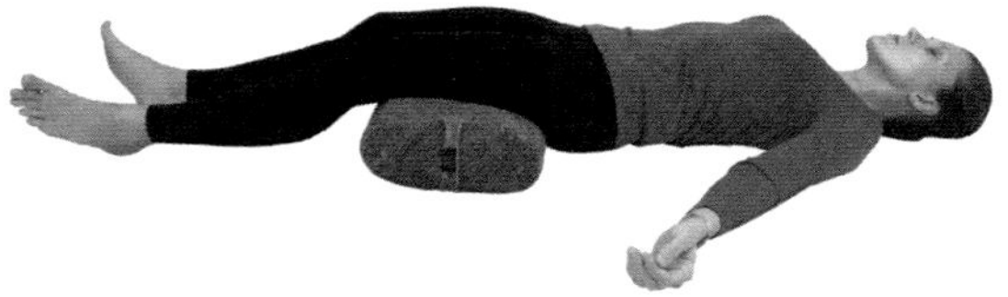

A lovely *Savasana* would fit well at the end of this sequence (with the bolster placed horizontally under your thighs, just above your knees, accompanied by relaxed breathing).

This simple routine does wonders for the spine, as well as digestion and the vagus nerve as it unravels the tension that comes from habitually rounding forward. It can provide sweet relief in those moments when we feel like we don't have time for more relaxation. If you are short on time, after the final restorative pose in the sequence just return to what is for you a more natural breath and slowly make your way to an upright seated position, then continue with your day. However, if you feel that you do have the time and you or your student/client needs extra healing time, follow the whole practice with seated diaphragmatic breathing and a short meditation.

PUSHAN MUDRA FOR DIGESTION

Like acupuncture and acupressure, *mudras* (energetic seals or gestures) are said to influence the flow of energy through the body, creating a circuit, as it were.

Pushan Mudra (the gesture of digestion) is a hand *mudra* used to activate *prana vayu* (the energy of receptivity), *samana vayu* (the energy of digestion and assimilation), and *apana vayu* (the energy of elimination). Unlike many other *hasta* (hand) *mudras* in which both hands are in the same position, the fingers of the right hand create a receptive position, while those of the left hand take a form that represents elimination.

Pushan is a solar deity whose work is to conduct souls to the afterlife. He also appears at times of transition in life, like marriage, relocation, or the birth of a child. Times that may be...well, hard to digest. As such, *Pushan Mudra* can be used to help us assimilate and process anxieties that may arise in new phases of life.

On a physical level, *Pushan Mudra*—which is associated with the stomach, liver, and gallbladder—is classically practiced as a means to relieve nausea, flatulence, and the after-effects of rich meals, though it is not meant to replace medical treatment. On emotional and mental levels, when times are anxious and changing and we need extra help to better digest life, hand *mudras* such as *Pushan* can be our "yoga on the go."

Classically, hand *mudras* are practiced for 45 minutes a day in 5-minute intervals (to balance the five elements), but any time you have can be beneficial. While you can enjoy this hand *mudra* in any body position, I like to practice in *Vajrasana* (Thunderbolt Pose, or kneeling with legs and feet together and sitting back on the heels) or *Bhadrasana* (Gracious Pose, a wide-kneeling posture with big toes touching) for additional stimulation to the digestive meridians.

Some experiences are definitely harder to digest than others and better physical digestion is a means to better digestion of life. Classic techniques like breath awareness combined with *Pushan Mudra* allow us to simply and subtly move through transitions on all levels of being.

Right-hand *mudra*

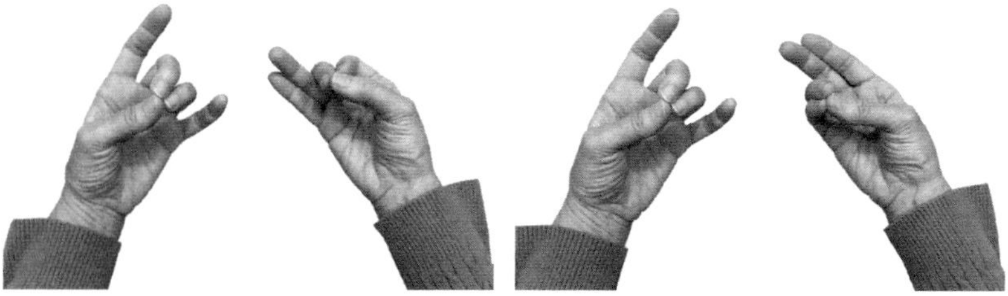

For upper gastro-intestinal tract issues such as reflux and belching:

Press the tips of your index and middle fingers to the tip of your thumb. Your ring and little fingers remain outstretched, your palm facing up.

For lower gastro-intestinal tract issues such as gas, bloating, or constipation:

Press the tips of your ring and little fingers to the tip of your thumb. Your index and middle fingers remain outstretched, your palm facing up.

Left-hand *mudra*

The left hand is the same for all gastro-intestinal issues:

Press the tips of your middle and ring fingers to the tip of your thumb. The index and pinky fingers remain outstretched, your palm facing up. (One of my daughters suggested that if you forget how to create this hand position, use the mnemonic "left looks like a llama.")

With the backs of your hands resting on the top of your thighs (in a place that doesn't create tension in your arms or shoulders), increase the pressure from your fingertips on the thumb on your inhalation and release the pressure a little on exhalation for a relaxing effect.

CHAPTER 11

The Breath with the Creative Process as a Path toward Fearlessness

I hear students and clients say that they forget to breathe. When asked why, fear often underlies this tendency—fear of doing a pose wrong, of not pleasing the teacher or therapist, of falling down. Once we can get over the hurdle that stopping the breath is not going to help, a change begins. And in that change of view, more freedom in creativity begins.

There is an exquisite birthing process that happens when ordinary movement becomes *asana*. It is that brief period when breath fully takes residence in the body—when we feel the breath as though it were luxuriating in the roll of our wrists, or the softness of our eyes. In that *asana*'s lifespan, there is cleansing, expansion, stillness, and sustenance. Aren't these qualities the building blocks for being fully alive?

Experiencing the artistry of yoga can be a process of allowing breath to evolve into a beautiful creative expression.

Just as an artist begrudgingly toils over a commissioned piece not to their liking, or a musician plays trite requests in quiet frustration, yoga practitioners can also make the practice of postures a colorless workout. Experiencing the artistry of yoga can be a process of allowing breath to evolve into a beautiful creative expression—a beauty that expands to fill the canvas of the mind and body.

When this happens, we're not just painting by numbers; we're seeing the clean surface and the frame into which life itself emerges.

In my work as a singer I often performed with musicians who technically played chords correctly, but it was a rare pleasure to create music among master players whose music would make me spontaneously weep and laugh with joy. I could hear the way these musicians were breathing as they played—at times effortlessly and rhythmically; at others, fiercely and intensely, punctuating phrases with a gushing exhalation. They played oblivious to the sounds of their powerful inhalations or sighing exhalations. They were so tuned into the music they were creating, it was as if they were breathing life into their instruments—infusing their art with a piece of their soul.

As a funny side note, master yogini Shiva Rea once told me I had an amazing ribcage while we were practicing a breath technique—a compliment I'll carry longer than most because it was so unexpected. Like many singers and horn players, my broad, mobile ribs have kept me from wearing tight bodices, but singing makes me forget disappointment about my wardrobe. Developing my diaphragm was never an intentional focus for me as a singer. The music was the priority and the mechanics of breath were not. Yet, through natural diaphragmatic breathing, I'd surprise myself by holding notes an impossibly long time—notes I was able to hold, not through willpower, but because of the *prana* (life force) generated through the creative process.

My husband and daughters are visual artists and, like my musician friends, the same creative process involving breath rhythm and tone happens in their work, especially during the editing process, where refinement and shading bring out texture and light. I notice that their breathing patterns become deep and audible, or that they change with the movement of the pen or brush. Many artists refer to their works as their "children," and the labor and delivery process are aided by the way they move the breath.

My paternal grandfather taught penmanship and created beautiful calligraphy. He was known to faint from holding his breath when he rendered a bird or created a document. Perhaps his breath retention, like *Kumbhaka* (a breath-control technique that focuses on retention), helped channel his life force into his work. However, unlike yogis (who have established practices in holding the breath), his cessation of breath caused him to lose consciousness rather than move into a higher state (although, curiously, he was considered to be a saintly man by many who knew him).

It is in times of focused breath practices (such as *Nadi Shodhana*, *Kapalabhati*, or *Ujjayi*) that my own ideas for a new class composition or fresh concepts for a writing project emerge. Then when I draw my attention to the sensation in my nostrils and smell the perfume of *prana shakti* (life force), my mind feels expansive. Ideas come unbidden and flow easily, like gifts. I try to encourage these insights to wait until the meditation's end, but they are often quite insistent. Conversely, when I'm laboring over an assigned piece, the ideas and breath are often choppy, merely functional, or joyless until I remember to breathe into the process.

When my husband and I named our yoga education center "Teach to Inspire," it was based on the dual meanings of the word "inspire," which are: 1) To fill (someone) with the urge or ability to do or feel something, especially to do something creative, and 2) To breathe in (air); inhale. Enchanted as we were with the name and the meanings behind it, this is far from an original concept. The recognition of the connection between the creative process and breath is recognized in scripture. For example, the breathing of life force is mentioned 15 times in the Bible alone, and more often in the *Bhagavad Gita*, the *Upanishads*, and the *Dhammapada*.

In my experience, what happens in the process of lovingly giving birth to a yoga practice or creative endeavor is initially a cleanse and nourish process. It brings us into the present; and in the now, fear and anxiety rarely exist. We begin by exhaling attachment to our old shape (the old shape of our bodies, emotions, or minds), while we inhale something higher (who we want to become). If we let go of who we were and what we have done before, the space is created for what we can become. Often the gift which we are searching for—the ease in the pose, the quieter mind, the clear idea, the vision or music—is not something we have to earn. Instead it comes to us by means of our creating space for it to blossom. We exhale to create space for life, God, *prana*, the higher mind, Nature, Love—call it what you will—and what fills the space is a better, freer version of ourselves.

Through our bodies we can experience the essence behind *pranayama*. What begins as simple, mechanical alternate nostril breath can become a tangible cleansing of energy channels (*nadis*). The pause to observe following *Bhastrika* practice delights us with a warm, tingling feeling—somewhat like a sweet blooming of flowers at our temples, or the sparkling of fireflies across our skulls. The sensation gently invites us into the preciousness of meditation. We sit in that space not because it is a harsh discipline but because we delight in the exploration. We are no longer practicing like new piano students with timers, but lingering like seasoned musicians, elated because life has given us a new piece to play.

Then from this lovely process of creating space for the new (which can happen thousands of times a day) comes phase two—which is shaped by what we receive and what we have the capacity to give. The unobstructed breath, which fills our practice, is of the receiving of not just oxygen, nitrogen, and carbon dioxide, but of *prana* itself. With this *prana*-filled breath, we have the capacity to inspire others. This lovely inspiring movement is what we see in the refined practices of master yogis and artists. Instead of strain, we see clear, meditative eyes and a body and heart in harmony. In that beauty, we are awakened to the potential of humanity in harmony with creation beyond our former association with anger, sorrow, and anxiety.

A PRACTICE FOR SHAPING POSTURES WITH BREATH

APANASANA (KNEE TO CHEST)

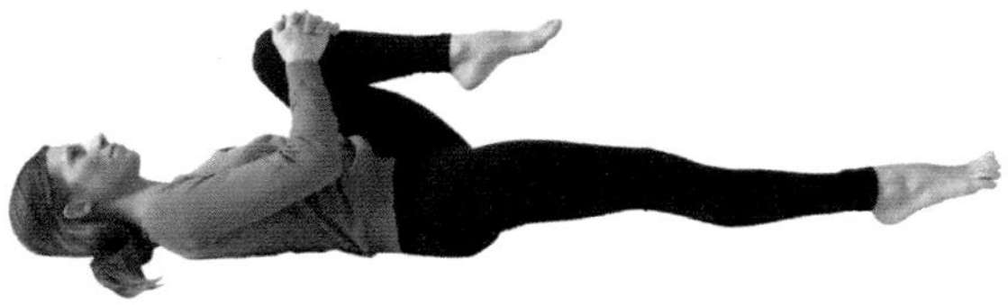

Start by warming your body with some reclining alternate knee *Apanasana*, squeezing your knee firmly to your abdomen on exhalation. Do this 10 times on each side.

SPINE CIRCLES

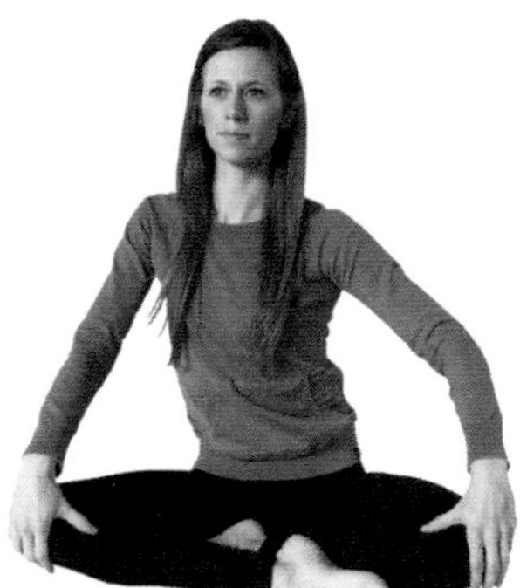

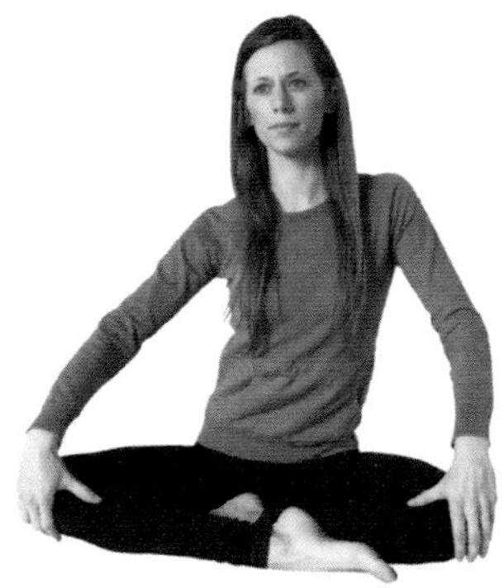

Come to *Sukasana* (Easy Posture). Hands on knees spiraling the spine. Inhale as chest moves forward and exhale as abdomen draws back.

Now you are ready to begin the slow deep stretches. Take at least 20 breaths in each pose. Feel the pose evolve with each expansion and contraction of the breath.

MAKARASANA (CROCODILE POSE) AND *PARSVA MAKARASANA* (SIDE CROCODILE POSE)

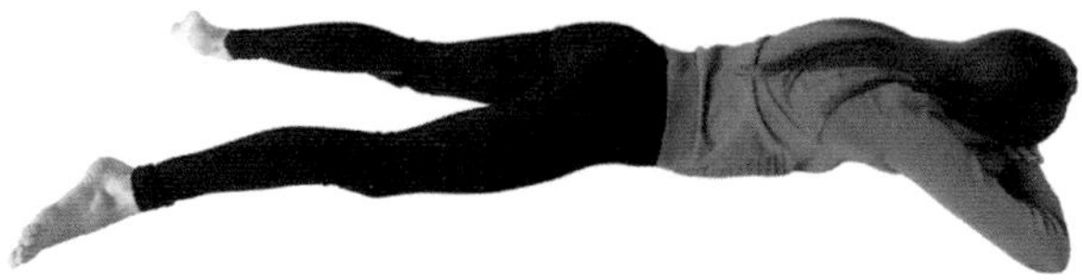

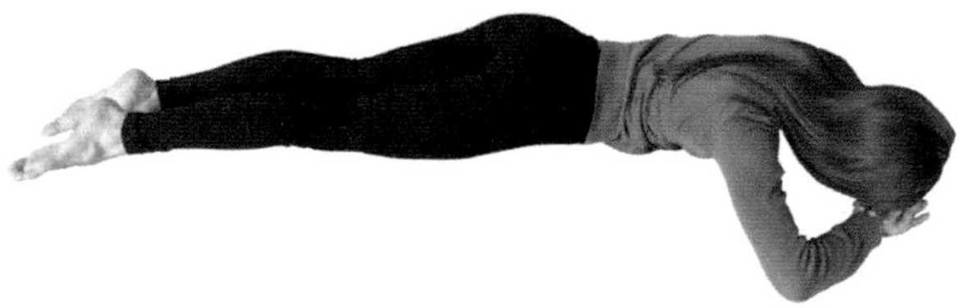

Makarasana is done prone, with your legs a comfortable distance apart and your forehead resting on your stacked forearms. Your upper ribs should be slightly away from the floor. Stay in this position for 10–20 breaths, allowing your breath to expand into your sides and the back of your torso.

To move into *Parsva Makarasana*, shift your upper body to the right and bring your left leg to join your right leg so that your body forms a prone arch. After 20 breaths, return to center and repeat on the other side.

PARIVRTTA JANU SIRSASANA (REVOLVED HEAD-TO-KNEE POSE)

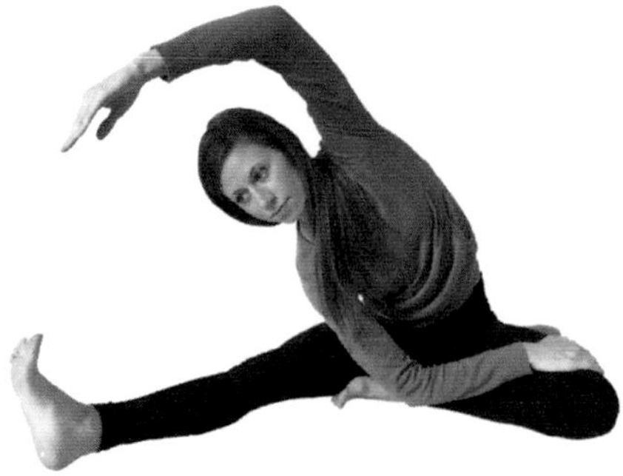

Start seated on the floor with legs wide and a slight elevation (folded blanket) of the sit bones and take the sole of your left foot in, toward your right inner thigh. You may be more comfortable sitting on a folded blanket, which will tip your pelvis forward and prevent your low back from collapsing.

With your spine still upright, rotate your chest toward your bent (left) knee on an inhalation and lift your ribcage up, away from your pelvis.

Take your right hand to your left thigh, exhale, and twist to the left, focusing the twist in your upper torso as you open through your chest and ribcage.

Inhale as you bring your left arm up, alongside your left ear. Exhale as you bend sideways to the right, pressing down into your bottom arm to allow your chest and face to rotate upward. Your right (straight leg) knee may need to bend a little if you'd like to try to link your left hand to your right outer foot. Alternatively, just enjoy the openness in your left ribs and allow your left arm to arc gently in line with your left ear. If it's in your practice to reach your right outer foot, you can bring your right hand over to join the left on either side of the foot. If you lose some of your rotation in doing so, or if your breath becomes ragged, return to your bottom hand reaching across the body.

Parivrtta Janu Sirsasana can evolve and expand with longer holds; 5–10 smooth breaths here may leave you feeling a sense of calm, or a "delightful buzz" (as I like to call it), which means the vagus nerve is telling your body that "everything is going to be just fine."

BHARADVAJASANA (BHARADVAJA'S TWIST POSE)

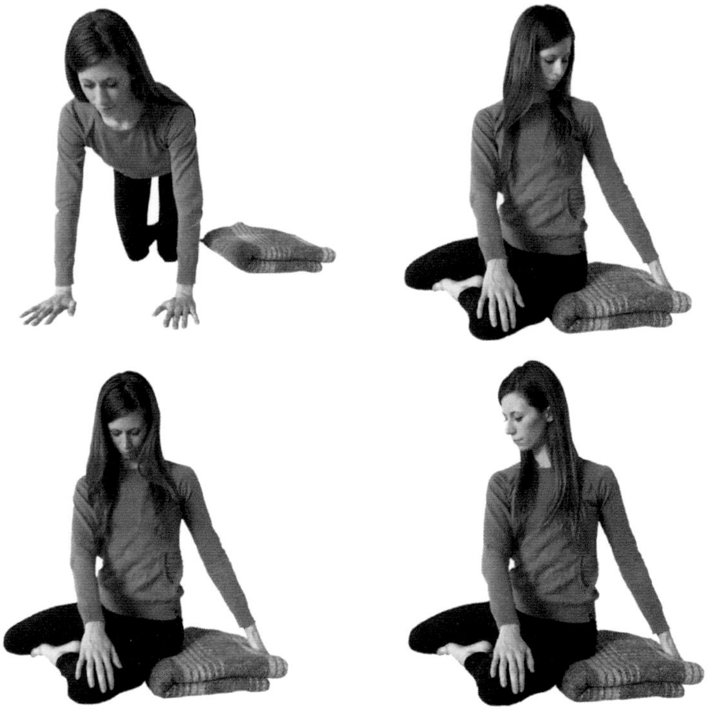

Lift through the crown of your head and revolve your torso to the right, taking your right hand toward the floor or a block, and your left hand to your outer right thigh.

Revolve your head to the right, then drop your chin and softly roll your head to the left. Stay for 5 breaths, then switch to the left side.

VIPARITA KARANI (LEGS UP THE WALL)

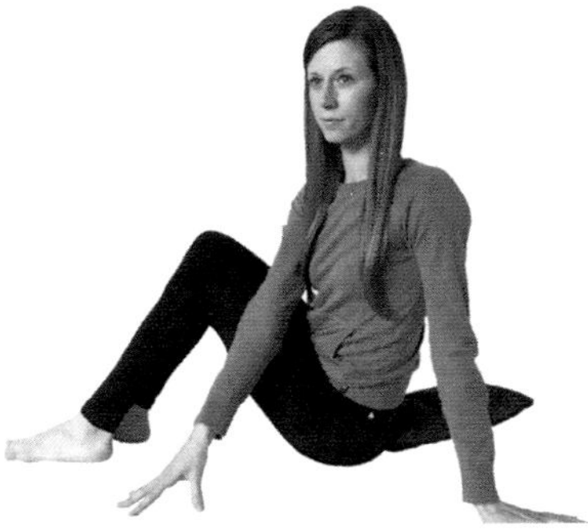

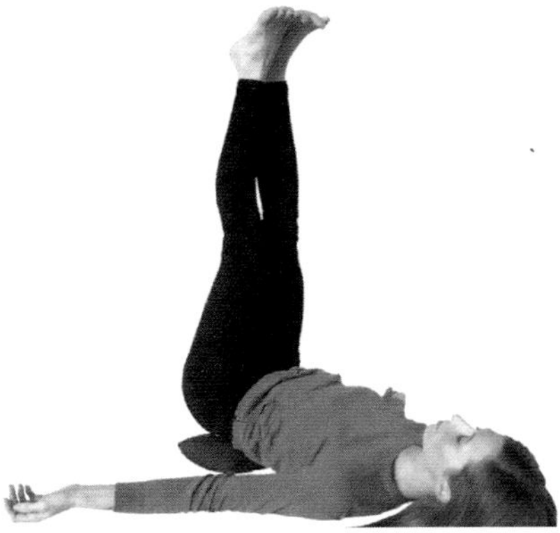

Sit with your right hip flush to a wall, then pivot your legs up the wall and scoot in until you are as close as possible. Lift your hips by pressing your feet to the wall and slide a bolster horizontally under your hips. Stay for 10 breaths.

Roll onto your side to come out of the position. Stay on your side for 5 breaths (your blood pressure may be lowered a bit and you'll want to avoid dizziness or the slight chance of a stroke).

SUPPORTED BACKBEND

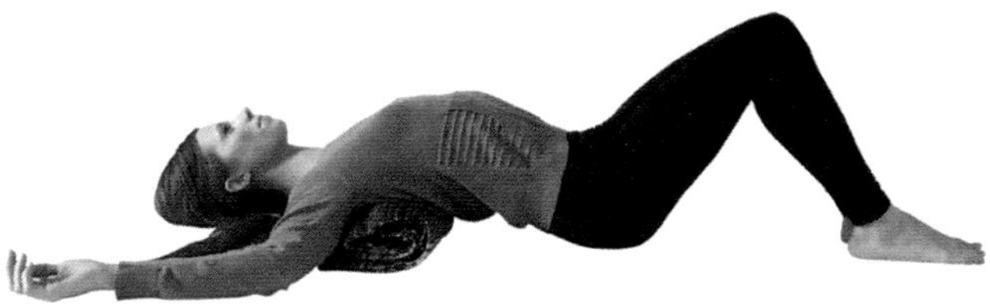

Lying on your back, place a rolled blanket horizontally behind your heart and extend your arms out to a T position behind the roll. Bend your knees, place your feet on the floor, and breathe around the pressure behind your shoulder blades, releasing tension in the thoracic spine. A good length of time to spend in the pose is 10 breaths.

PSOAS TWIST

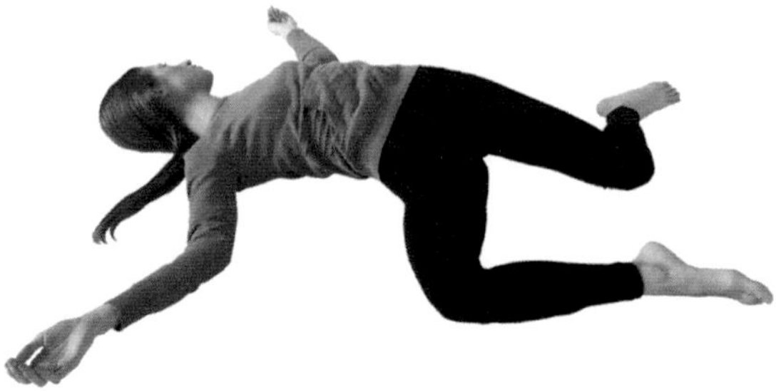

Lie on your back with your knees bent, your feet mat-width apart, and your arms extended in a wide V with your palms facing up. Take both your knees gently to the right on an exhalation as your head turns left for a long extension of your torso. After 20 breaths, repeat on the left side.

BALASANA (CHILD'S POSE)

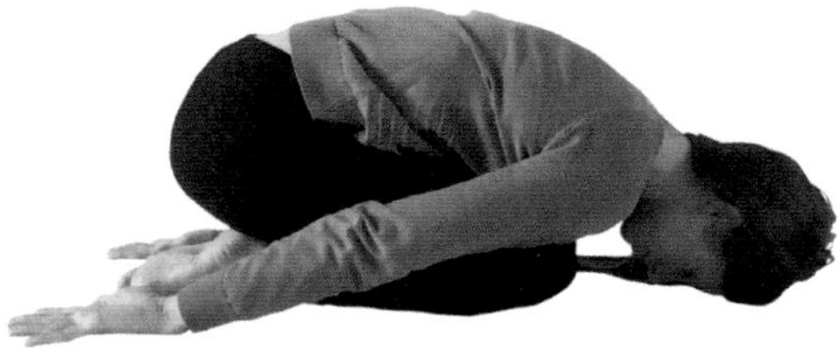

Kneeling in a Forward Fold, breathe into the back of your body for around 3 minutes.

PARIVRTTA BALASANA (TWISTED CHILD'S POSE)

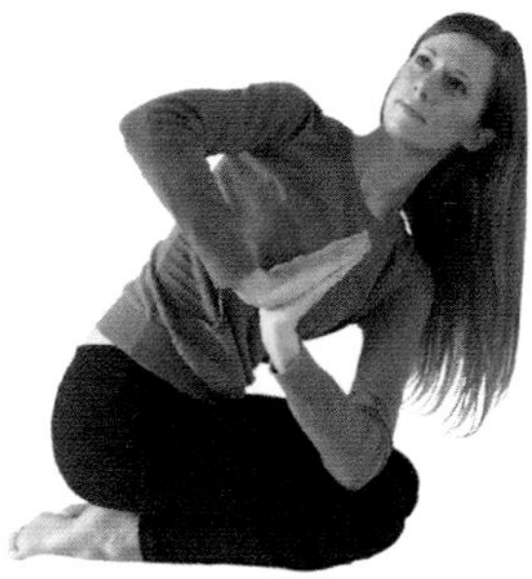

From Child's Pose, bring your left elbow to your outer right knee, and your hands into a prayer position. Then relax and melt your left shoulder toward your outer right knee. Breathe around the deep twist for 5 breaths. Repeat on the other side.

SALAMBA BADDHA KONASANA (QUEEN'S POSE)

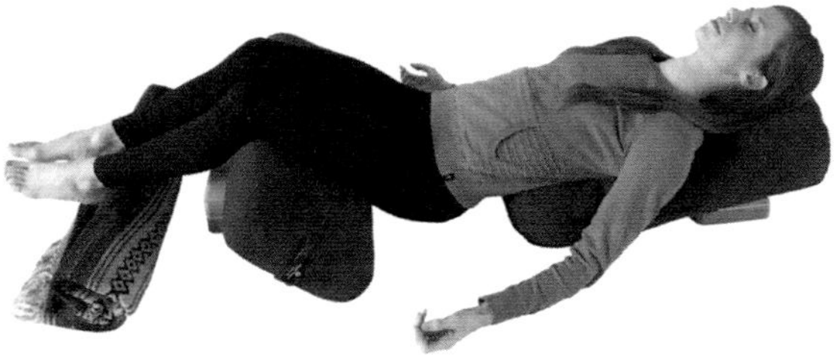

Tilt one bolster vertically with a block to support your lumbar spine up to your head (like a recliner). Use a second bolster propped horizontally at an angle under your thighs, with your knees relaxed outward. Use a blanket to support your head further if needed or a rolled blanket under your ankles. Use a blanket to cover the body, and use a focused awareness to relax the body from the crown of the head to the soles of the feet and then back to the head.

NADI SHODHANA (ALTERNATE NOSTRIL BREATHING)

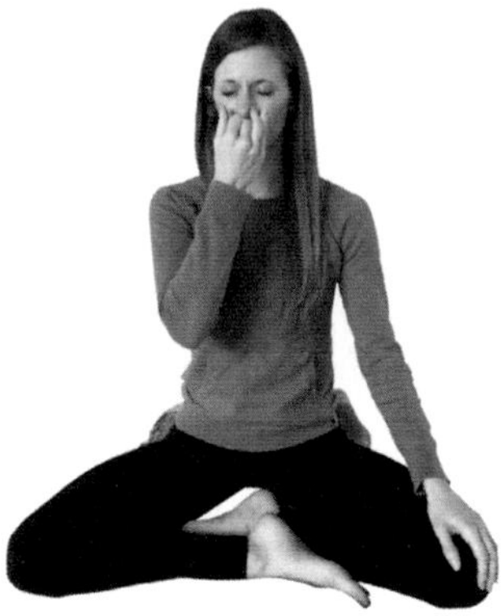

Allow the spine to lengthen so that the head, neck, and trunk are aligned. Gently close the eyes.

Begin by taking a full, deep inhalation followed by a slow, gentle exhalation. In this way, practice several rounds of diaphragmatic breath.

Bring the right hand into *Vishnu Mudra* by folding the tips of the index and middle fingers inward until they touch the palm at the base of the right thumb. During this practice, you will alternately use the right thumb to close the right nostril and the right ring and pinky fingers (together) to close the left nostril.

Use the right thumb to lightly close the right nostril. Exhale through the left nostril. Keeping the right nostril closed, inhale through the left nostril and deep into the belly.

Next, use the ring and pinky fingers of the right hand to close the left nostril and simultaneously release the right nostril. Pause gently at the bottom of the exhalation.

Keeping the left nostril closed, inhale once again through the right nostril, then again use the right thumb to close the right nostril as you release the left nostril. Exhale through the left nostril.

This completes one round of *Nadi Shodhana*. Repeat this alternating pattern for several more rounds. It is important that the breath remain slow, gentle, fluid, and relaxed throughout the practice.

PRANA DHARANA (LIFE FORCE CONCENTRATION)

Choose from one of the following Methods:

Method 1

PHASE 1

Come to an upright seated posture. Start with a circular *Nadi Shodhana*:

Slowly inhale through your left nostril and exhale through your right nostril 3 times. Rest for 3 breaths, then inhale through your right nostril and exhale through your left nostril for 3 rounds. Rest in breath awareness after round 3.

You can do multiple cycles of this, but just one is often pretty effective if you're short on time. This helps sensitize the area of the nostrils to which we are bringing attention.

PHASE 2

Relax into abdominal breath, feeling the nuances of the breath dropping down below your ribcage. Then without changing the relaxed way you are breathing, bring awareness to the feeling of the breath moving through your chest.

Draw your attention to the passage of air through your throat; at this point feel the coolness of the breath entering your body and the warmth of the breath leaving your body.

Now feel the subtlety of the breath in your nostrils, brushing in and out.

Then bring awareness to only the upper part of your nostrils, following a line up the interior nostrils to the point between your eyebrows.

Draw that line deeper into your head as though forming an arc from the tip of your nose to the center of your head (the mid-brain around the hypothalamus, the thalamus, the pituitary, and pineal area (the *pranic* hub)). Maintain a steady flow of breath and focus your attention on its subtlety. A *mantra* like *so-ham*, or a personal *mantra* can accompany the breath if desired.

Method 2

Phase 1

Begin with a breath practice. *Bhastrika* (Bellows Breath) is often effective in waking up nasal sensitivity. This is done with strong exhalation and inhalation emanating from the abdomen, with abdominal contraction on the exhalation, at a pace that allows for complete inhalation and exhalation (often around 50 rounds per minute).

If you feel dizzy or the Bellows Breath feels uncoordinated, you can use *Nadi Shodhana* above.

Phase 2

Drop into relaxed diaphragmatic breathing with attention focused on the bottom rim of your nostrils (the area closest to your lips).

Move your attention to the outer rim of each nostril, as though the breath were flaring your nostrils on the inhalation and relaxing the nostrils on the exhalation

Bring your attention to the sensations of the breath brushing the interior rim of your nostrils and septum.

Now, feel the breath along the upper nasal membranes, gathering more and more sensitivity to both directions of the breath, both in and out, and lift that awareness as though it was sweeping the frontal lobe of your brain. After sitting with this consciousness of breathing for a few minutes, focus your mind on an inspirational or scriptural passage or *mantra* to help hold your attention.

Method 3

Phase 1

This time, use the same weight of inhalation and exhalation as in *Bhastrika* (see Method 1, Phase 1 above), with abdominal contraction on the exhalation, for an alternate nostril practice. This practice is called *Surya Bhedi* (Sun-Piercing Breath).

Block the flow of breath through your left nostril by pressing lightly right below the nose cartilage with your left ring finger, then breathe through your right nostril: Exhale-inhale-exhale-inhale.

Now switch sides, blocking the flow through your right nostril with your thumb, and exhale-inhale-exhale-inhale through the left nostril. Do this 10 times on both sides.

After 10 rounds, take a long inhalation through your right nostril. Hold briefly and release slowly. Repeat on the other side.

Phase 2

Begin with long, relaxed abdominal breathing until the rhythm of the breath is steady and the inhalation and exhalation are balanced in length and quality.

Focus on the temperature in your right nostril as your breath moves in and out of it.

Refine your awareness down to the finest line of where you feel coolness on the way in and warmth on the way out.

Locate the point where the breath changes temperature.

Now do the same in your left nostril, really refining a sense of location of temperature change and minute refinement.

Bring your awareness to both nostrils, attempting to feel very balanced between both hemispheres of your brain and a sense of brain synergy for your meditation practice—even the attempt to feel this balance can be very refreshing.

CHAPTER 12

Heal the World by Living Courageously

Twelve Step Programs encourage people to move through the steps and to become sponsors and helpers to others who are also on the path to recovery from living in addiction and shame.* Being someone's mentor means knowing that how you live your life matters to someone you are mentoring and is a mutual aid to recovery. Similarly, becoming active in a community can make a difference when feeling insecure and intimidated; it is a way of first testing the water and then swimming out to help those in need and helps us become stronger swimmers. Activism which is also *Karma* Yoga is a viable spiritual path, one that helps make us stronger and more resilient against the fear around us.

"I've been watching you on social media. You are an activist," a forthright friend commented about my sometimes blunt commentary on human, civil, and animal rights. "That is rare for a yoga teacher. Most seem to think they can *Om* it all away." This not an uncommon assertion—a lot of people don't know how many yoga teachers are actively involved in helping groups and individuals overcome the anxiety, depression, and rage that plague our world, especially at this time in history.

Others in the yoga community often respond similarly to my petitioning and protest. They say things like, "The world reflects only that which we choose to hear; stay above the noise of the media."

* See https://www.aa.org, for example.

"I take long breaks from outside input to keep my consciousness clear. It might be good for you, too." "Take your frustration and fears to the mat! Process it there."

To those yogis, with their reasonable perspectives and honorable intentions, I say, "Thank you. But that's not my path."

I might have known there would be another path for me when I retreated to *ashram* life in a spiritual community a few years ago—only to discover that the *ashram* was now also a retreat center where various groups of differing perspectives and spiritual traditions shared space. I had thought I was ready to snuff out my activist candle and begin kindling my *agni* (internal or spiritual fire), as *Vedic* tradition suggests for those past the age of childrearing, in order to gracefully begin moving toward old age. But as hard as I blew on the candle, it continued to burn, with my desire to alleviate suffering and to right injustices pouring kerosene on the flame. Spirited conversations about human dignity and justice found their way to the community dinner table. Retreatants arrived from all parts of the world and all walks of life, with stories that made me cry and want to help. The passion for effecting positive change thrust me again into the world of petitions and protests. I provided financial support for organizations I believed in, and spoke from my heart when opportunities arose. My rekindled activism seemed spurred on by the words of the wise teachers I'd encountered over the years and by my long-standing meditation practice. "Let's do something of merit in this lifetime!" said the voice of my soul, intending something more than contemplating my navel.

My teacher, Eknath Easwaran, walked with Gandhi at a very frightening time in history in the salt marches to protest British rule in India. Easwaran fully understood the need to effect change in his lifetime. Studying with him in the 1980s, I watched him encourage the *ashram* children to work to save elephants from poachers. He created a program to bring deeper meaning in life to seniors, continually interacting with those who promoted peace globally. *Laurel's Kitchen*, inspired by Easwaran, was among the first successful vegetarian cookbooks. As did his role model, Mahatma Gandhi, Easwaran spoke of activism as a lifestyle. He believed that living a kinder, more conscious life would gradually change the world around us, and he saw vegetarianism as an important piece of that low environmental impact, good *karma* lifestyle.

The 80s were a rebound from the Vietnam War, with less protest and more introspection. We were dubbed the "Me" generation (akin to what I see in much of today's "It's just me and my mat" yoga). What Easwaran taught gave me hope. I was too young for the radical fury of the 60s, and hip but quiet Berkeley, California, where I lived, was mellow in the aftermath of its experience with social activism. But Easwaran was awake to the suffering of the planet, and he saw the enormous potential in using the energy generated in meditation to heal the world.

Easwaran's now classic translation and commentary on the *Bhagavad Gita—The End of Sorrow: The Bhagavad Gita for Daily Living, Vol I*—offers this rallying appeal:

> A family of two or three or four will not satisfy us; we will want a whole continent for our family, as Gandhiji had. When Mrs. Gandhi was asked how many children she had, her reply was, "I have four, but my husband has four hundred million." As meditation deepens and self-will becomes less, we come to regard everyone as our own; if they have problems, it is our privilege to live for helping them to solve those problems. When at last we regard the entire world as our family, we will be enabled to draw upon the vast reservoir of love and wisdom lying unsuspected in all of us.[1]

The tradition of *Karma* Yoga, the path of selfless service, long predates Mahatma Gandhi, and crosses the imaginary barriers between East and West. We can see the flame of social activism in the works of Jesus Christ and in the saints of the Judeo-Christian traditions. Within my lifetime, Martin Luther King, Jr. opened racial doors, and Mother Teresa of Calcutta modeled the caring and honoring of the poor as a way to level society's hierarchy. Nobel Peace Prize winner Malala Yousafzai inspires us with her exceptionally brave support of women's education in Pakistan. Like Arjuna, hero of the

Bhagavad Gita, these are spiritual warriors. Some might feel instead that a life of quiet contemplation is the most "yogic," but for those who are called to activism, a life sequestered in a monastery will never be satisfactory. The Malalas and the Martin Luther Kings would not have changed the course of human history through lives of only contemplation.

The inspirational saint Mother Maria Skobtsova wrote these words prior to her death at the Ravensbrück concentration camp:

> The way to God lies through love of people. At the Last Judgment, I shall not be asked whether I was successful in my ascetic exercises, nor how many bows and prostrations I made. Instead I shall be asked, did I feed the hungry, clothe the naked, visit the sick and the prisoners. That is all I shall be asked. About every poor, hungry, and imprisoned person the Savior says, "I was hungry and thirsty; I was sick and in prison." To think that He puts an equal sign between Himself and anyone in need... I always knew it, but now it has somehow penetrated to my bones. It fills me with awe.[2]

Putting an equal sign between ourselves and others—the deep truth of such *karmic* service takes one's breath away.

Gandhi, through non-violent activism, brought centuries of oppressive rulership to an end. He never actually said, however, "Be the change you wish to see in the world." This was a convenient abbreviation of what he actually said, which takes more thoughtfulness: "If we could change ourselves, the tendencies in the world would also change. As a man changes his own nature, so does the attitude of the world change towards him… We need not wait to see what others do."[3]

It seems to me that Gandhi was saying: Do your *asana* and *pranayama* practice, and build your meditation to a steady fire—a fire that brings the kind of clarity that doesn't ask for approval or require conformity but sees what this life is meant to be.

For my life, that means service. It means activism. My path is to work for peace where there is violence. Peace comes by sitting together in unity to help bolster each other and dispel fear, whether in meditation or in protest, and by volunteering and standing with like-minded organizations to oppose those who would harm others. Donating money and voting and petitioning for legislative change can also bring peace. Meditation and prayer can, at one and the same time, both fuel and soften the action. Without meditation, I might burn in the fires of righteous opposition. Tempering that wildfire is what Gandhi's words bring to mind: "Change your nature," so that your humanitarian words and efforts become clearer, more persuasive, and more effective.

The *Karma* yogi's path is to work for peace where there is violence.

There is injustice, and there is human suffering and so much fear. The children, the old, the poor, and the mentally ill are dishonored every day. I could try to justify it with the argument that all is in order and the *karmic* wheel is rolling. But rationalizing suffering does not make it go away, and I need to do something. I can't *Om* it all away. My *dharma*, my spiritual path, is to sit to still my mind. And then to take a stand.

Just as with the final of the 12 steps—"Having had a spiritual awakening as the result of these steps, we tried to carry this message to those who need them, and to practice these principles in all our affairs"[4]—applying our efforts to assuage fear and oppression in others helps us to find our inner hero and get on with our own healing.

Seeing the Bluebird, Remembering Our Fearless Selves

When my girls were small, much time was spent in nature. My oldest, Emily, would guide her younger twin siblings. "See the bluebird, Paige?"

"Oh, they have a nest!" Paige would exclaim. Blythe would often be distracted by reflections in the water or insects in the bark of the tree.

"Look, you'll miss it!" Emily would say, gently taking Blythe's chin in hand and turning her face to see the nearly missed moment.

Delight would spread over Blythe's face when she spotted her favorite birds.

As someone who offers yoga, my time is spent this way. People come into training, or classes, or therapy sessions expecting a set of poses, a predictable script to offer to others or heal their own ills; instead, what we can give them is an arrow, a whiff of a fragrance, or a tilt of the chin that allows each of them their own moment of awareness. Only their own insights can give them the ability to move forward bravely.

In observing the students who have gone through our yoga school, it seems that this often occurs around the 100-hour mark of a teacher training. The vastness of yoga strikes them, and they start noticing the interconnection between all aspects of the practice—the limbs, the paths, *koshas, vayus, doshas*—and the utter hugeness of all that is yoga. And often, there is a sense of being overwhelmed: "I can't teach this! I may have to drop out of training!" That's when I know they have seen the bluebird. The ego has taken the necessary hit, and perhaps the teacher-in-training sees their new role: a humble tour guide pointing out the attractions with which they are familiar. A tour guide doesn't need to know the underlying geological formation of the Royal Gorge, or be able to recount the biography of every Renaissance painter in Florence. Having a deep, joyful connection with, and enthusiasm to explore, the area is what makes an effective tour leader—one who will stimulate other minds and hearts, and, when needed, point them in the direction of teachers with more understanding. (Here, again is the "Billy Goat Gruff" process: "No, don't eat me, my brother is much bigger!" is somewhat akin to "Go study with my teacher.")

In a public class, the "bluebird moment" often comes halfway through the class when we have thinned the exoskeleton of stress and fear, and a moment's pause arises. "Listen to your breath, do you notice how it is clear?" There are half smiles or nods. "How's your shoulder feeling?" we might ask as the student departs. The student's expression says, "What shoulder? I felt what yoga does." Aloud they say, "Better." In the context of a yoga class, or even a single *asana*, the recognition of just one breath can open a student's eyes to the *rasa* (the underlying juice of practice). Maybe they came for fitness but got a peek at something much bigger.

In Yoga Therapy sessions, expectations for results are particularly high. The Yoga Therapist's role is to uncover the body's habits and movement patterns that are at the root of the issue, and to then help the client unwind these old familiar patterns. The client's eyes are opened when they realize that all of their movement is yoga—not just what they do on the mat. One client of mine recently laughed, "When I wanted a private session, I thought you would teach me how to perform full King Dancer Pose, but instead I learned to walk!" Every client has to understand for themselves what subtle movements, breath patterns, and life skills can change their course.

In the *Bhagavad Gita* (2.54), Arjuna asks *Sri* Krishna, "Tell me of the man who lives in wisdom, ever aware of the Self, O Krishna; how does he talk, how does he sit, how does he move about?"[5] Arjuna has become aware of the deep layers and wants to see more. He has tilted his head to the perfect angle to see the goal, to walk around in a wise way, to be aware of the higher Self always. Arjuna wants to live in the state of fearlessly understanding why he came to this point and to behave wisely at all times, not just have the momentary glimpse.

The bluebird is fleeting for most of us. You see it, and clarity is yours; the threads connect and you see what work lies ahead. Then you leave teacher or Yoga Therapy training, and initial discouragements like small class attendance or lack of clients or payment darken your perceptions. You leave the public class vowing to start a home practice, to attend class regularly, and to hang out with people with similar goals. And then your children get the chickenpox, or you lose your job, and simply making it through the day becomes the top priority. Or the "aha" moments of a great Yoga Therapy session are lost when, in the midst of daily life, you forget the breathing or subtle alignment cues that previously served as a guiding light. But you saw the bluebird, and you aren't going to forget that. You looked at yoga and saw into its bottomless depths briefly, an ocean of knowledge so deep that it will take lifetimes to explore, but something changed. The Sanskrit word *smarana* (remembering who we really are) describes the sighting of the elusive bird, the clearing of the water, that thing we are looking for.

With regular practice, bluebirds become a familiar sight and they show up everywhere: in a breath at a stoplight, in a late evening walk, in the smile of a friend. And they are still present in the midst of illness, a messy divorce, or the death of a loved one—perched on top of our deepest fears.

Sri Krishna responds to Arjuna:

> He lives in wisdom
> Who sees himself in all and all in him,
> Whose love for the Lord of Love has consumed
> Every selfish desire and sense-craving
> Tormenting the heart. Not agitated
> By grief nor hankering after pleasure,
> He lives free from lust and fear and anger.
> Fettered no more by selfish attachments,
> He is not elated by good fortune
> Nor depressed by bad. Such is the seer.[6]

The word "seer" hits a resounding note. Someone who sees—sees without prompts and reminders, without tilting their head at an angle, or squinting just so. Seeing the underlying meaning, the beauty of the hidden bluebird, we need not look any further since we have found the source of joy.

Learning to Radiate Joy to Counter the Darkness

I'd like to share an example outlining a daily practice for self-healing taking our wellness beyond our yoga mat and dinner table, and in doing so, helping a fearful world that needs more people who are well and conscious.

Teachers of the Sikh tradition state that relaxation is the highest wisdom stemming from recognition of what we don't need, and that we don't have to chase the demons of fear and darkness and the concerns of being pulled downward in some way. For many of us the tug back into the fray of combating demons is strong, and a "blissed out" *Savasana* is hard-earned or nibbled away by doubts about our safety if we "let go."

There is a relaxation that comes from moving deeply inward and cultivating calm in ever more subtle layers. This is the type we most likely encounter in a yoga class and is effective for many. Another kind of relaxation is experienced after a genuine belly laugh, hearing a moving piece of music, or giving a gift from the heart. To understand these different types of relaxation, one can look to the different movements of *prana* (vital energy) throughout the body, known as *vayus*. The "moving inward" type of relaxation involves *samana vayu* (energy moving inward toward the center) and *apana vayu* (energy directed downward, i.e. grounding and settling), while the belly-laugh release involves *udana vayu* (energy uplifted) and *vyana vayu* (expanding outward). The idea that one can relax into a state of openness and brightness may be new (as we often tend to associate relaxation with grounding and turning inward), but relaxation practices that include *udana*- and *vyana*-focused visualizations can prove helpful, particularly when we're feeling tired or depressed. A Sikh sage once said that anything that can give you relaxation is God, so why not explore a method that may allow you, or a client, a relaxation that could help you find that state?

I would like to offer a *Savasana* particularly suited for morning practice or for times of sadness, when you need an energetic lift. If you are a teacher, you could read it to your class. If practicing on your own, you could record yourself reading the relaxation, or have someone read it to you. If you practice it often, you will likely commit it to memory.

SAVASANA FOR AN ENERGETIC LIFT

Begin by giving yourself permission to be truly comfortable. Cover your body, making sure that you're warm enough. Place a folded blanket under your head and a bolster under your thighs for more comfortable alignment of your back. Relax your arms about 12–16 inches from your sides, with your legs about mat-width apart.

Establish an easy awareness of the breath, and simply enjoy its rhythm, tone, and texture. Notice how the breath changes and adapts its movement to your relaxing body.

Bring your attention to your solar plexus (the upper central abdomen), and see if you can feel the warmth in this area—perhaps visualizing the sun there: *Surya, Surya, Surya*. Allow that warm radiance to begin a slow expansion outward to your navel, heart, and ribs. Take 3 slow, deep breaths, as though fanning the flame. Then expand the circumference of the rays of that sun to include your pelvis, the sides of your torso, and up to the notch of your throat. Take 3 slow breaths, encouraging warmth and light. Now, expand the brightness to include your jaw, upper arms, and extending down to your knees. Take 3 breaths, visualizing healing and ease in the ever-widening circle. The radiant circle includes the top of your head, and extends outward to your fingers and toes, as you breathe away any tension or effort.

Return to your solar plexus. Allow the sun at that center to radiate healing light and life outward through your toes, fingertips, and the crown of your head. See your practice as one of healing for all those around you. Your own inner peace is a gift of peace for all. Take several breaths, making them slow and deep.

Now, bring your attention to the tip of your nose, and sense the cool temperature of your breath as it moves in and the warm temperature as it moves out. Then focus your attention on only your right nostril, bringing your awareness to the fine line along which you feel the temperature of your breath, and the exact point where you feel the change in temperature. Remain at that point for 5 breaths. Repeat the same process in the left nostril for 5 breaths.

Finally, repeat the process in both nostrils together for 5–10 breaths, noticing how becoming more aware brings a tangible ease across your forehead and temples. Refine your awareness of the subtle, sweet expansion in your mind, radiating clarity through all your thinking processes. From your eyebrow center, emanate kindness and wisdom to all sentient beings.

As you slowly begin to move back into an awareness of your physical body, allow for a playful exploration. Stretch as though from a nap on a beach, awakening to a wonderful day ahead. Yawn and reach and wiggle. Roll to your right and smile.

Gently press yourself up to a seated posture—moving, with joy, into seated meditation if you wish.

Living Fearlessly Doesn't Mean Living Painlessly

While we hope that we can live in a "no pain, no pain" state, this is often what propels us into addiction in the hope of avoiding unpleasantness altogether.

Kundalini teacher Guruprem Khalsa, in an interview with Tommy Rosen, speaks in a voice reminiscent of the Buddha: "Pain is the currency of transformation, spend it wisely."[7]

Often, finding the usefulness of the fear of pain is what sets us toward our greater purpose. Ask many who are in recovery or who have experienced grief where they would be without the process. Ask them about the ways in which they've helped others out of their own excruciating life experiences through that process.

What comes out of surviving suffering, fear, and sorrow is a resilience born of pain, and a *hookum*—a message from your soul that says, "I have a special task for you."

The Goal of Yoga Therapy

In his book, *BodyMindCORE*, Rolfer and movement therapist Noah Karrasch talks about a common question among those working in a field related to healing the body/mind: "How do we get our clients to stand tall and move and breathe more fully from the core?"[8] In the Yoga Therapy room this is such an individual process that we often feel like Sherlock Holmes, tracing the place or places of stricture and finding ways to release the movement habits that are keeping our client stuck.

We start at the physical level and work on posture of course, but yoga asks us to look at living from our full stature, and so often the lack of self-worth or shame underlying posture can be addressed just by helping the body recognize its potential. Addressing the physical is not always just for the physical's sake—Yoga Therapists start at the physical level because we're multidimensional beings (as master Yoga Therapist and founder of the American Viniyoga Institute Gary Kraftsow would say), but even at that layer we can still do deeper work/work on the other layers of our being.

The idea of moving from a deeper awareness of the body is often lost in a lot of shape/alignment-focused *asana* as we contort the body in order to achieve extreme poses. Regaining a fluid gait and letting the whole body be responsive to a standing pose can help re-educate the body to move in a way that *supports* (as opposed to moving in a way that *distorts*). This process serves to remind us to move from the core of our being—who we actually are—rather than moving for the sake of achievement of shapes measured by someone else's concept of "doing it right."

The breath in Yoga Therapy becomes progressively deeper to heal the nervous system, and also to heal the mind. The more we learn about the subtleties of the breath, the more we establish a connection to the subtleties of the mind and can begin to unravel the *samskaras* that are shackling us to repeat the same old behaviors. As the breath is, so is the mind.

It's no wonder people often leave a Yoga Therapy session feeling euphoric; they are reminded that they are more than a body that moves, pivots, and breathes from a point of pain and fear. They are literally centered.

As Bessel van der Kolk listened to one of his patients in a therapy session—a Vietnam War veteran who didn't want to take medication to stop his recurring nightmares—the man wanted to have nightmares to become a living memorial to those who died in combat. I've heard similar stories of retaining symptoms to honor a traumatic event. People hold trauma in their hearts and bodies as well as their brains.

It's not simply cognitive; trauma gets stuck in the body and nervous system. That's why talk therapy is often ineffective. We may be able to say that a frightening experience is no longer in the present but we feel that it is and feel that it is still harming us.

Those who do not experience PTSD are able to rewrite history with a more positive perspective, while those who experience ongoing symptoms of trauma cannot. It is always in the now.

Van der Kolk believes yoga to be therapeutic and that, like EMDR, it can help sufferers to get back into their bodies and feel what is truly happening now.

During many fearful times of our lives we have the desire to grab the reins and steer life to go our way. But in my experience, forcing an outcome has had limited to no success. Below is a set of affirmations—prayers if you will—that can be very helpful in walking forward with less anxiety about the future.

1. *Let go of the outcome.* This is the most difficult act of *Ishwara Pranidhana* (surrender) when affirmed daily or even better each time anxiety or frustration eventually takes hold.

2. *Know that the solution exists.* We all have had the experience of worrying and stressing, only to be surprised by the outcome—often it's far better than we expect.

3. *Express gratitude for the solution.* If you've let go of the outcome, it doesn't matter what that solution is, does it? Just be grateful that the solution exists.

4. *Stop fretting.* It's done, and your role is just to walk through the open door.

Glossary

abhaya	Fearless.
Abhaya Mudra	Gesture of fearlessness; *mudra* literally means seal.
Abhinivesha	Fear of death.
Abhyasa	Regular practice.
agni	Fire.
Agni Sara	Fire essence.
ahimsa	The principle of non-violence.
Akanda mandalakaram visvam vyaya vyavasthitam Trailokya manditam yena mandalam tat sadasivam	The invocation prayer for the *mudra* connoting the non-dual concept of the presented universe and the perceiving self, or the microcosm in the macrocosm. *Mandala* is the geometric expression which enables the seeker to direct the individual constitution toward evolution.
Ananda	Bliss.
Anjali Mudra	A gesture or seal of reverence; prayer gesture.
annamayakosha	The physical layer; literally, the sheath made of food.
Apanasana	Knees to chest.
apana vayu	*Apana* is the *prana vayu* that involves the downward and outward flow of energy from the body. *Apana vayu* governs the outward flow of energy on the breath, with digestive elimination, and with menstruation.
asana	A posture in which a practitioner sits or moves.
ashram	A hermitage; a spiritual community or retreat.
Ashtanga	Eight limbs.

Atman	The higher Self.
Aum	A sacred sound and spiritual icon.
Ayurveda	The science of life or lifespan, Yoga's ancient sister science.
Balasana	Child's Pose.
bandhanan	From bondage.
bandhas	Locks, usually referring to the "body locks" in *Hatha* Yoga. Specific *bandhas* are: *Mula Bandha*, contraction of the perineum; *Uddiyana bandha*, contraction of the abdomen into the ribcage; *Jalandhara Bandha*, tucking the chin close to the chest.
Bhadrasana	The Gracious Pose; sitting between the heels with knees wide.
Bhagavad Gita	"The Song of the Lord"; name of a Hindu scripture which contains the instructions of Lord Krishna.
Bharadvajasana	Twist Pose dedicated to the sage Bharadva.
Bhastrika	Bellows Breath.
bhavana	An intentional meditation technique to invoke a certain feeling or quality.
bhaya	Fear.
Bhuta Shuddhi	A meditation preparation to "cleanse the elements."
bija mantra	Sacred seed word containing potency.
Brahmari Breath	Bumblebee or Humming Breath.
brahmin	A caste or class in Hinduism specializing as priests, teachers, and protectors of sacred learning across generations.
chakra	A "wheel" or center of energy.
Chaturanga	Four-Limbed Staff Pose; a yoga push-up.
Dhammapada	A collection of sayings of the Buddha in verse form and one of the most widely read Buddhist scriptures.
dharana	Concentration, the first stage of meditation; the sixth limb in Patanjali's yoga system.
dhyana	Meditation; the second stage of meditation in Patanjali's yoga system.

dosha	One of three energies, or constitutional types in *Ayurveda.*
Gita	"The Song"; a shorter term for the *Bhagavad Gita.*
guru	Spiritual teacher.
Guru Stotram	A prayer glorifying a spiritual teacher.
ha	Sun/solar (masculine).
Hare Krishna	*Hare* addresses divine energy; *Krishna* means he who is attractive to everyone.
Hare Rama	*Hare* addresses divine energy; *Rama* means joy.
hasta	Hand.
Hatha Yoga	The physical practices. *Hatha* means force; in syllables, it means sun and moon.
Hridaya Abhaya Mudra	Fearless Heart gesture or seal.
hukam	In Sikhism, represents the goal of becoming in harmony with the will of God and thus attaining inner peace.
Ishwara Pranidhana	Surrender to Divine plan.
japa	Repetition of a *mantra.*
Jnani (*jna* "to know")	One who follows the path of knowledge and study.
kama	Selfish desire, greed; sometimes personified as *Kama-deva*, "god of desire."
Kapalabhati	Skull-Shining Breath.
kapha	The *Ayurvedic dosha* of earth and water.
kaphic	Having attributes of *kapha dosha*; cool, heavy, and moist.
karma (*kri* "to do")	Action; former actions which lead to certain results in cause and effect relationship.
Karma Yoga Therapy	Selfless service as a path to healing.
Katha Upanishad	The most widely known of all the *Upanishads. Katha* is a style of storytelling and *Upanishad* means legend.
koshas	Sheath or layer that covers the Self (*Atman*).

kriya (*kri* "to do")	Actions done with a specific intention. In Kundalini yoga there may be many intentions behind certain movements, breath practices, chanting and their duration. Kundalini *kriyas* often involve vigorous "breath of fire," dynamic movements and require stamina, pushing us a bit past our comfort zone and often making us forget our obsessions with the busy mind. Initially, the purpose of performing such *kriyas* is to open blockages in the energetic system—at a chakra, for instance—or maybe to improve lymphatic drainage on the physical level. In latter practice the *kriyas* are said to take one to the next level of spiritual development.
Kumbhaka	The pause between an inhale and exhale.
kundalini	Primal energy that can affect changes in consciousness.
Kundalini Shakti	Primal energy recognized as the divine feminine.
Kundalini Yoga	A style of yoga practice associated with Yogi Bhajan and influenced by Shaktism and Tantra schools.
Maha Mrityunjaya Mantra	Conqueror of Death prayer. Also known as the *Tryambakam.*
Mantra	A verse of the *Rig Veda.*
Makarasana	Crocodile Pose.
mala	A garland or necklace of 108 beads used to count prayers or *mantras.*
manipura chakra	City of jewels energetic center located at the navel/solar plexus area; the third major chakra.
Manomayakosha	Composed of *manas* or mind; said to be constituted of the mind (*manas*) along with the five sensory organs.
mantra	A sacred sound or name.
mantram	Used alternately (often regionally) for the word *mantra.*
Matsyasana	Fish Pose; a pose dedicated to the sage Matsya.
Moorcha	Swooning Breath.
mrtyormukshiya	To free, liberate from death.
mudra	A seal or gesture of the body.
Mula	Bandha Root Lock; a lift of the pelvic floor.

nadi	A channel or flow of energy through the subtle body.
Nadi Shodhana	Channel cleansing.
Namaskara	Salutation.
niyamas	Positive duties or observances; the second limb of Patanjali's yoga system.
Om Eim Saraswatyei Swaha	Salutations and Eim (a seed mantra) to Saraswati, so be it!
pancha vayus	The five airs or winds.
Pandit	A title for an honored scholar.
Parivrtta Balasana	Revolved Child's Pose.
Parivrtta Janu Sirsasana	Revolved Head-to-Knee Pose.
Parsva Makarasana	Side Crocodile Pose.
pitta	Fire/water *dosha.*
Prachardhana	A breath practice from the *Yoga Sutras.*
prana	Life force.
Prana Dharana	Life force concentration.
pranamayakosha	The sheath of energy covering the higher Self.
prana shakti	The life force recognized as the divine feminine.
prana vayu	A wind or movement of life force.
pranayama	Breath practices.
Pranic Vayus	The winds or movements of life force.
pratyahara	Withdrawal of the senses; the fifth limb of Patanjali's yoga system.
preya	That which is pleasant.
Purvottanasana	Eastward Facing Stretch or Upward Plank Pose.
Pushan Mudra	A gesture for digestion named for a Vedic solar deity.
pushti	A well-nourished condition, thriving, prosperous, fullness of life.
Qigong	A Chinese system of physical exercises and breathing control related to *Tai Chi.*
Raja Yoga	The royal path of meditation.
rama	Joy.
rasa	Essence, flavor, juice.
sadhana	Daily spiritual practice.

Salamba Baddha Konasana	Supported Bound Angle Pose.
samadhi	Enlightenment; the eighth limb of Patanjali's yoga system.
samana vayu	"Balancing Air or Wind"; one of the five *vayus* that make up *prana*. Believed to exist in the abdomen with the navel as its energy base, and oversees the digestion of everything from food to thoughts.
samskara	A personality trait conditioned over one or many lives: a mental and behavioral pattern; a latency or tendency within the mind which will manifest if given the proper environment or stimulus.
Saraswati	Goddess of knowledge, music, art, wisdom, and learning. She represents that river of creativity that flows through us.
Sarva Trikhanda Mudra	*Sarva* means "all or everything," *Trikhanda* means "consisting of three parts," and *Mudra* means "seal."
satsang	A spiritual gathering or discourse.
sattwic	Pertaining to an attribute (*guna*) that has elevating quality of nature.
Savasana	Corpse Pose.
sheetali	A cooling breath practice through a curled tongue.
shloka	A type of sung verse in Sanskrit.
shreya	That which is beneficial.
Sitali (alternate spelling for *sheetali*) *Pranayama*	Cooling type of breath practice.
smarana	Remembering who we are.
so-ham	A *mantra* meaning "I am That."
spanda	The sacred shiver.
Spandana	A therapeutic practice with origins in *tantric* Shaivism that shakes the body.
Sri (pronounced *Shree*)	An honorarium connoting both respect and beauty.
Srividya Yantra	An ancient and influential school of Goddess-centered *Shakta Tantrism*. A *yantra* is a visual *mantra*.
sugandhim	Sweet fragrance, fragrant.
Sukhasana	Easy posture.
Surya Bhedi	Sun-Piercing Breath.
sushumna	"Very gracious" or "kind"; also the name for the central *nadi* in the body.

swadhisthana	"Her own dwelling place"; the second *chakra* located at the sacrum.
Swami	A yogi who has been initiated into a religious monastic order.
Tadasana	Mountain Pose.
Tai Chi	An internal Chinese martial art practiced for both its defense training and its health benefits.
Tandava	The sacred dance of Shiva.
tantra	In the past, meant loom; also specifically, the warp thread that dresses the loom and gives support to the fabric formed by the moving shuttle or, in a rug, the individual knots. It now refers to a lineage tradition passing on practices to enable spiritual growth.
tapas	"Discipline"; the third of Patanjali's *Niyamas*. Derived from the root Sanskrit verb "tap," which means "to burn" and evokes a sense of "fiery discipline" or "passion."
tejas	Inner radiance, fire, or illumination; can be classified as a type of energy, vitality, or charisma.
tha	Moon or lunar (feminine).
Thoppukaranam	Hands to Ears *Kriya*. Also known as "Superbrain Yoga."
tridoshic	Pertaining to all three *doshas*: *vata*, *pitta*, and *kapha*.
Trikhanda Mudra	Three-part gesture or seal.
trikhanda	Having three parts.
tryambakam	The three-eyed one, Siva.
udana vayu	Upward-moving energy
Ujjayi Breath	Victorious Breath.
Upanishads	"Legends"; refers to Hindu sacred treatises written in Sanskrit c. 800–200 BC, expounding the *Vedas* in predominantly mystical and monistic terms.
urvarukam iva	Like the cucumber or melon.
vairagya	Detachment from material life.
Vajrasana	Thunderbolt Pose.
vam	A seed *mantra* (*bija*) for the second *chakra*.

vardhanam	One who nourishes, strengthens, causes to increase (in health, wealth, well-being); who gladdens, exhilarates, and restores health; a good gardener.
Vasisthasana	Side Plank Pose named for the sage Vasistha.
vata	The *dosha* of wind and air.
vatic	Pertaining to *vata dosha*; it is light, dry, and mobile.
vayus	Winds or airs.
Vedanta	Ancient spiritual philosophies and one of its broadest, based on the *Vedas*, the sacred scriptures of India.
Vedic	Relating to the *Veda* or *Vedas*.
vijnanamayakosha	The wisdom sheath that overlies the Self. *Vijnanamaya* encompasses intuition and intellect.
vinyasa	Flowing postures connected with breath.
Viparita Karani	Inverted Action or Legs Up the Wall Pose.
vipassana	To see things as they really are; one of India's most ancient techniques of meditation.
viveka	Discernment or right understanding.
vrittis	A fluctuation in consciousness, like wave patterns from a stone thrown in the water.
vyana vayu	One of the five subdivisions of *prana*. *Vyana* means "outward-moving air" and *vayu* means "wind."
yajamahe	We worship, adore, honor, revere.
yamas	Restraints or ethical rules; the first limb of Patanjali's yoga system.
Yin (in Chinese philosophy)	The passive female principle of the universe. In yoga it means long, slow, passive stretch.
Yoga Sutras	A collection of aphorisms written by Patanjali, these "threads" (as *sutra* translates from Sanskrit) of wisdom offer guidelines for purposeful living, leading to life's goal of higher consciousness.

Notes

Chapter 1

1. Aamodt 2012.
2. Ito et al. 1998.
3. Kerr 2015.
4. Manning-Schaffel 2017.
5. Bhartrihari 1976.
6. Ferriss 2007.
7. Kaminoff 2009.
8. Leitzell 2008.
9. Gates 2017.
10. Porges 2007.
11. Assaraf 2016.
12. Lazar et al. 2000.
13. Farb et al. 2007.
14. Streeter et al. 2010.
15. Selvamurthy et al. 1998.
16. Boston University School of Medicine 2007, 2017.
17. Kiecolt-Glaser et al. 2010.
18. Sengupta 2012.
19. Easwaran 2001, p.116.
20. Post 2005.
21. Easwaran 2007.
22. Hanh 1987.

Chapter 2

1. Treault 2017.
2. Tigunait 2013.
3. Van der Kolk 2011.
4. Thondup 1996.

Chapter 3

1. Yehuda et al. 2000.
2. Easwaran 2008.
3. Rossen 2014.
4. Easwaran 2005, p.156.
5. Quoted in Conner 2011.
6. Easwaran 2014.
7. Easwaran 2009, p.41.
8. Easwaran 2009, p.42.
9. Tigunait 2008, p.66.
10. Olson et al. 2006.
11. Yuede et al. 2009.
12. Easwaran 1984, p.89.

Chapter 4

1. Hanson 2009, p.3.
2. Hanh 1991, p.10.
3. Brown 2012.
4. Chödrön 2002.
5. Verma and Kumar 2016.

Chapter 5

1. Streeter et al. 2007.
2. Treault 2017.
3. EurekaAlert 2010.
4. Van der Kolk 1994.
5. Van der Kolk 2014.

Chapter 7

1. Selye 1976.
2. Van der Kolk, Brown and van der Hart 1989; Scaer 2001.
3. Van der Kolk 1994.
4. Yalom and Yalom 2010.
5. Buczynski 2014.
6. HealthyPsych 2017.
7. Quoted in Read-Smith 2017.
8. Seigneur 2013; Woods 2004.
9. Masullo and Tripodi 2016.
10. Howard 2013.

11. Marich 2015.
12. Van der Kolk 2014.
13. Menendez and Williams 2007.
14. Chandrasekran, Rajesh, and Srinivasan 2014.

Chapter 8

1. Quoted in Rodriguez 2012.
2. Morriss-Kay 2010.

Chapter 10

1. Quoted in Gostica 2016.
2. Quoted in Gostica 2016.
3. Millera and Newberry 2010.
4. Caffrey 2013.
5. Kaswala 2013.
6. Keefer and Blanchard 2001.
7. Frøkjaer et al. 2016.
8. Suarez et al. 2010.

Chapter 12

1. Easwaran 1984.
2. Marshall and Mosher 2011, p.8.
3. Gandhi 1999, p.241.
4. Alcoholics Anonymous 1952, p.106.
5. Easwaran 1984, p.103.
6. Easwaran 1984, pp.105–111.
7. Khalsa 2017.
8. Karrasch, White, and Buri 2017, p.27.

References

Aamodt, S. (2012) "An Interview with John Cacioppo: The Science of Loneliness." *Being Human: How Social Isolation Changes the Brain and Behavior.* Accessed on 10/03/17 at www.beinghuman.org/article/interview-john-cacioppo-science-loneliness.

Alcoholics Anonymous (1952) *Twelve Steps and Twelve Traditions.*

Assaraf, J. (2016) "Webinar." 12 August 2016. Accessed on 9 March 2018 at https://m.facebook.com/story.php?story_fbid=10154452969453658&id=76062578657&_rdr.

Bhartrihari, V.-S. (1976) *The Hundred Verses on the Renunciation.* Translated by Swami Madhavananda. Calcutta: Advaita Asharama.

Boston University School of Medicine (2007) "Study finds yoga associated with elevated brain GABA levels." 22 May. Accessed on 9 March 2018 at www.bu.edu/news/2007/05/22/study-finds-yoga-associated-with-elevated-brain-gaba-levels.

Boston University School of Medicine (2017) "Yoga Can Help Reduce Symptoms of Depression." Accessed on 9 March 2018 at www.bumc.bu.edu/busm/2017/03/08/yoga-can-help-reduce-symptoms-of-depression.

Brown, B. (2012) *The Power of Vulnerability: Teachings on Authenticity, Connection, & Courage* [CD]. Louisville, CO: Sounds True.

Buczynski, R. (2014) "Rethinking Trauma: The Third Wave of Trauma Treatment." *National Institute for the Clinical Application of Behavioral Medicine.* Accessed at http://www.nicabm.com/rethinking-trauma-the-third-wave-of-trauma-treatment-2 on 17 April 2018.

Caffrey, M. (2013) "Restorative Yoga Better Than Stretching for Trimming Subcutaneous Fat in Overweight Women." *American Journal of Managed Care.* Accessed on 9 March 2018 at www.ajmc.com/journals/evidence-based-diabetes-management/2013/2013-1-vol19-sp7/restorative-yoga-better-than-stretching-for-trimming-subcutaneous-fat-in-overweight-women.

Chandrasekeran, A., Rajesh, S. and Srinivasan, T. (2014) "Effect of repetitive yogic squats with specific hand position (Thoppukaranam) on selective attention and psychological states." *International Journal of Yoga* 7, 1, 76–79.

Chödrön, P. (2002) *When Things Fall Apart: Heart Advice for Difficult Times.* London: Element.

Conner, J. (2011) *My Soul Pages: A Companion to Writing Down Your Soul.* San Francisco, CA: Conari Press.

Easwaran, E. (1984) *The End of Sorrow: The Bhagavad Gita for Daily Living, Vol I, Chapter 3.* Petaluma, CA: Nilgiri Press.

Easwaran, E. (2001) *The Constant Companion: The Thousand Names of Vishnu.* Tomales, CA: Nilgiri Press.

Easwaran, E. (2005) *Words to Live By: Short Readings of Daily Wisdom.* Tomales, CA: Nilgiri Press.

Easwaran, E. (trans.) (2007) *The Upanishads.* Tomales, CA: Nilgiri Press.

Easwaran, E. (2008) *God Makes the Rivers to Flow, Sacred Literature of the World.* Tomales, CA: Nilgiri Press.

Easwaran, E. (2009) *Essence of the Upanishads: A Key to Indian Spirituality.* Tomales, CA: Nilgiri Press.

Easwaran, E. (2014) "The Way of Non-Attachment." *Yoga International.* Accessed on 9 March 2018 at https://yogainternational.com/article/view/the-way-of-non-attachment.

EurekaAlert (2010) "Surprise: Scientists discover that inflammation helps to heal wounds." Federation of American Societies for Experimental Biology. Accessed on 9 March 2018 at www.eurekalert.org/pub_releases/2010-10/foas-ssd100410.php.

Farb, N., Segal, Z., Mayberg, H., Bean, J., McKeon, D., Fatima, Z. and Anderson, A. (2007) "Attending to the Present: Mindfulness Meditation Reveals Distinct Neural Modes of Self-Reference." Oxford Academic. Accessed on 9 March 2018 at https://academic.oup.com/scan/article/2/4/313/1676557.

Ferriss, T. (2007) "The 4-hour work week." CNNMoney.com, 5 September. Accessed on 9 March 2018 at http://money.cnn.com/2007/05/04/magazines/fsb/4_hour_week.fsb/index.htm.

Frøkjaer, J.B., Bergmann, S., Brock, C., Madzak, Farmer, A.D., Ellrich, J. and Drewes, AM. (2016) "Modulation of Vagal Tone Enhances Gastroduodenal Motility and Reduces Somatic Pain Sensitivity." *PubMed 4,* 592–598.

Gandhi, M. (1999) *The Collected Works of Mahatma Gandhi, Vol 13, March 12, 1913–December 25, 1913.* New Delhi: Publications Division Government of India.

Gates, R. (2017) "Meditations from the Mat and along the Road to Recovery." Recovery 2.0 Conference with Tommy Rosen, December 2017.

Gostica (2016) "Our second brain—the gut feels, acts and recalls more than the head." *Gostica,* 25 October 2016. Accessed on 12 March 2018 at https://gostica.com/spiritual-nutrition/second-brain-gut-feels-acts-recalls-head.

Hanh, T.N. (1987) *Being Peace.* Berkeley, CA: Parallax Press.

Hanh, T.N. (1991) *Peace Is Every Step: The Path of Mindfulness in Everyday Life.* New York: Bantam Books.

Hanson, R. (2009) *Buddha's Brain: The Practical Neuroscience of Happiness, Love, and Wisdom.* Oakland, CA: New Harbinger Publications.

HealthyPsych (2017) "Trauma and PTSD." Accessed on 9 March 2018 at https://healthypsych.com/trauma-and-ptsd.

Howard, M. (2013) "Part I: Trauma training should be mandatory for yoga teachers." *Huffington Post,* 17 May. Accessed on 12 March 2018 at https://www.huffingtonpost.com/margaret-howard/part-i-trauma-training-sh_b_3290291.html.

Ito, T.A., Larsen, J.T., Smith, N.K. and Cacioppo, J.T. (1998) "Negative information weighs more heavily on the brain: The negativity bias in evaluative categorizations." *Journal of Personality and Social Psychology 75,* 4, 887–900.

Kaminoff, L. (2009) Talk given at The Breathing Project, New York.

Karrasch, N., White, R. and Buri, E. (2017) *BodyMindCORE Work for the Movement Therapist: Leading Clients to CORE Breath and Awareness.* London: Singing Dragon.

Kaswala, D., Shah, S., Mishra, A., Patel, H. *et al.* (2013) "Can Yoga be Used to Treat Gastroesophageal Reflux Disease?" *International Journal of Yoga 6,* 2, 131–133.

Keefer, L. and Blanchard, E.B. (2001) "The effects of relaxation response meditation on the symptoms of irritable bowel syndrome: results of a controlled treatment study." *Behaviour Research and Therapy 39,* 7, 801–811.

Kerr, M. (2015) *SCREAM: Chilling Adventures in the Science of Fear.* Philadelphia, PA: PublicAffairs.

Khalsa, G. (2017) *Finding the True Path of Recovery: Moving from the Head to the Heart.* [Podcast]

Kiecolt-Glaser, J., Christian, L., Preston, H., Houts, C., Malarkey, W.B., Emery, C.F. and Glaser, R. (2010) "Stress, Inflammation, and Yoga Practice." *Psychosomatic Medicine 72,* 2, 113–121.

Lazar, S., Bush, G., Gollub, R., Fricchione, G., Khalsa, G. and Benson, H. (2000) "Functional brain mapping of the relaxation response and meditation." *NeuroReport.* Accessed on 9 March 2018 at http://prsinstitute.org/downloads/related/spiritual-sciences/meditation/FunctionalBrainMappingoftheRelaxationResponseandMeditation.pdf.

Leitzell, K. (2008) "The Other Brain Cells: New Roles for Glia." *Scientific American.* Accessed on 9 March 2018 at www.scientificamerican.com/article/the-other-brain-cells.

Manning-Schaffel, V. (2017) "A fondness for fear: Why do we like to be scared?" *NBC News,* 23 October. Accessed on 9 March 2018 at www.nbcnews.com/better/health/fondness-fear-why-do-we-be-scared-ncna812661.

Marich, J. (2015) "An Open Letter from a Trauma Therapist to Yoga Teachers: 12 Simple Ways to Make Your Classes More Trauma-Informed." *Elephant Journal.* Accessed on 9 March 2018 at www.elephantjournal.com/2015/01/an-open-letter-from-a-trauma-therapist-to-yoga-teachers-12-simple-ways-to-make-your-classes-more-trauma-informed.

Marshall, D. and Mosher, L. (eds.) (2011) *Prayer: Christian and Muslim Perspectives.* Washington, DC: Georgetown University Press.

Masullo, L. and Tripodi, M. (2016) "Crawling towards a map of the brain." *eLife 5,* e15438.

Menendez, D.S. and Williams, P. (2007) *Becoming a Professional Life Coach: Lessons from the Institute for Life Coach Training.* New York: W.W. Norton & Company.

Millera, M. and Newberry, R. (2010) "Microanatomy of the Intestinal Lymphatic System." *Annals of the New York Academy of Sciences 1207,* Suppl 1, E21–E28.

Morriss-Kay, G. (2010) "The Evolution of Human Artistic Creativity." *Journal of Anatomy 216,* 2, 158–176. Olson, A.K., Eadie, B.D., Ernst, C. and Christie, B.R. (2006) "Environmental enrichment and voluntary exercise massively increase neurogenesis in the adult hippocampus via dissociable pathways." *Hippocampus 16,* 3, 250–260.

Porges, S.W. (2007) "The Polyvagal Perspective." *Biological Psychology 74,* 2, 116–143. http://doi.org/10.1016/j.biopsycho.2006.06.009

Post, S. (2005) "Altruism, Happiness, and Health: it's good to be good." *International Journal of Behavioral Medicine 12,* 2, 66–77.

Read-Smith, M. (2017) "Trauma and science." Accessed on 12 March 2018 at www.markreadsmith.com/trauma-and-science.

Rodriguez, T. (2012) "Creativity predicts a longer life: The trait of openness improves health through creativity." *Scientific American,* 1 September. Accessed on 12 March 2018 at https://www.scientificamerican.com/article/open-mind-longer-life.

Rosen, T. (2014) *Recovery 2.0: Move Beyond Addiction and Upgrade Your Life.* Carlsbad, CA: Hay House.

Scaer, R.C. (2001) "The neurophysiology of dissociation and chronic disease." *Applied Psychophysiology and Biofeedback 26,* 1, 73–91.

Seigneur, E. (2013) "Ask a neuroscientist: How to train your brain." *NeuWrite West Blog,* Stanford Neurosciences Institute, 13 August. Accessed on 12 March 2018 at https://neuroscience.stanford.edu/news/ask-neuroscientist-how-train-your-brain.

Selvamurthy, W., Sridharan, K., Ray, U.S., Tiwary, R.S. *et al.* (1998) "A new physiological approach to control essential hypertension." *Indian Journal of Physiology and Pharmacology 42*, 2, 205–213.

Selye, H. (1976) *Stress in Health and Disease.* Boston, MA: Butterworths.

Sengupta, P. (2012) "Health Impacts of Yoga and Pranayama: A State-of-the-Art Review." *International Journal of Preventative Medicine 3*, 7, 444–458.

Streeter, C.C., Jensen, J.E., Perlmutter, R.M., Cabral, H.J. *et al.* (2007) "Yoga Asana Sessions Increase Brain GABA Levels: A Pilot Study." *The Journal of Alternative and Complementary Medicine 13*, 4, 419–426.

Streeter, C., Whitfield, T., Owen, L., Rein, T. *et al.* (2010) "Effects of Yoga Versus Walking on Mood, Anxiety, and Brain GABA Levels: A Randomized Controlled MRS Study." *Journal of Alternative and Complementary Medicine 11*, 1145–1152.

Suarez, K., Mayer, C., Ehlert, U. and Nater, U.M. (2010) "Psychological stress and self-reported functional gastrointestinal disorders." *The Journal of Nervous and Mental Disease 198*, 3, 226–229.

Thondup, T. (1996) *The Healing Power of Mind.* Boston, MA: Shambhala Publications.

Tigunait, R. (trans.) (2008) *The Pursuit of Power and Freedom.* Honesdale, PA: Himalayan Institute Press.

Tigunait, R. (2013) "Living Tantra, Part 7: Advanced Prana Dharana." *Yoga International.* Accessed on 9 March 2018 at https://yogainternational.com/article/view/living-tantra-part-7-advanced-prana-dharana.

Treault, N. (2017) "The Power of Breath." *Awesome Neuroscience.* Accessed on 9 March 2018 at www.nicoletetreault.com/single-post/2017/04/14/The-power-of-breath.

Van der Kolk, B. (1994) "The Body Keeps The Score: Memory & the Evolving Psychobiology of Posttraumatic Stress." *Harvard Review of Psychiatry 1*, 5, 253–265.

Van der Kolk, B. (2011) "The vagus nerve, emotions and the difficulty with mindfulness practices." *Healing From the Freeze.* Accessed on 9 March 2018 at https://healingfromthefreeze.wordpress.com/2011/08/18/the-vagus-nerve-and-the-difficulty-with-mindfulness.

Van der Kolk, B. (2014) "Restoring the Body: Yoga, EMDR, and Treating Trauma." *On Being.* Accessed on 9 March 2018 at https://onbeing.org/programs/bessel-van-der-kolk-restoring-the-body-yoga-emdr-and-treating-trauma. [Podcast]

Van der Kolk, B.A., Brown, P. and van der Hart, O. (1989) "Pierre Janet on post-traumatic stress." *Journal of Traumatic Stress 2*, 4, 365–378.

Verma, S. and Kumar, K. (2016) "Evidence based study on super brain yoga and its application on alpha E.E.G. in adolescence." *ResearchGate 2*, 4, 40–46.

Woods, C.G. (2004) "Neuroscience. Crossing the midline." *Science 304*, 5676, 1455–1456.

Yalom, V. and Yalom, M-.H. (2010) "Peter Levine on Somatic Experiencing." Accessed on 17 April 2018 at https://www.psychotherapy.net/interview/interview-peter-levine.

Yehuda, R., Bierer, L., Schmeidler, J., Aferiat, D.M.S.W., Breslau, I.M.A. and Dolan, S.B.A. (2000) "Low Cortisol and Risk for PTSD in Adult Offspring of Holocaust Survivors." *The American Journal of Psychiatry 157*, 8, 1252–1259.

Yoga International (2013) "Purify Your Chakras, Part 4: How to Practice Bhuta Shuddhi." Accessed on 9 March 2018 at https://yogainternational.com/article/view/purify-your-chakras-part-4-how-to-practice-bhuta-shuddhi.

Yuede, C.M., Zimmerman, S.D., Dong, H., Kling, M.J. *et al.* (2009) "Effects of voluntary and forced exercise on plaque deposition, hippocampal volume, and behavior in the Tg2576 mouse model of Alzheimer's disease." *Neurobiology of Disease 35*, 3, 426–432.

Subject Index

Author Index